Pharmacological Treatment of Tics

Pharmacological Treatment of Tics

Andrea E. Cavanna
University of Birmingham

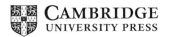

CAMBRIDGE
UNIVERSITY PRESS

University Printing House, Cambridge CB2 8BS, United Kingdom

One Liberty Plaza, 20th Floor, New York, NY 10006, USA

477 Williamstown Road, Port Melbourne, VIC 3207, Australia

314–321, 3rd Floor, Plot 3, Splendor Forum, Jasola District Centre,
New Delhi – 110025, India

79 Anson Road, #06–04/06, Singapore 079906

Cambridge University Press is part of the University of Cambridge.

It furthers the University's mission by disseminating knowledge in the pursuit of
education, learning, and research at the highest international levels of excellence.

www.cambridge.org
Information on this title: www.cambridge.org/9781316649398
DOI: 10.1017/9781108186599

First published 2020

Printed in the United Kingdom by TJ International Ltd, Padstow Cornwall

A catalogue record for this publication is available from the British Library.

Library of Congress Cataloging-in-Publication Data
Names: Cavanna, Andrea E., author.
Title: Pharmacological treatment of tics / Andrea E. Cavanna.
Description: Cambridge, United Kingdom ; New York, NY : Cambridge University Press, 2020. | Includes
bibliographical references and index.
Identifiers: LCCN 2019056917 (print) | LCCN 2019056918 (ebook) | ISBN 9781316649398 (hardback) |
ISBN 9781108186599 (ebook)
Subjects: LCSH: Tic disorders – Chemotherapy. | Tic disorders – Diagnosis.
Classification: LCC RC552.T5 C38 2020 (print) | LCC RC552.T5 (ebook) | DDC 616.8/3061–dc23
LC record available at https://lccn.loc.gov/2019056917
LC ebook record available at https://lccn.loc.gov/2019056918

ISBN 978-1-316-64939-8 Paperback

....

To the patients met along the journey – Adam, Adrian, Akindele, Alan, Alex, Alexander, Alisha, Andrew, Anita, Antonia, Anthony, Ashish, Ashley, Barbara, Belinda, Benjamin, Bruce, Callum, Casey, Catherine, Cavan, Charlotte, Charles, Christiana, Christopher, Christy, Claire, Clive, Cody, Colin, Connor, Cristian, Daniel, Danny, Darren, Dawn, Dean, Dedeh, Dylan, Dzak, Eadyn, Edward, Elinor, Elizabeth, Ellie, Emma, Erika, George, Georgia, Georgina, Gerry, Glen, Gordon, Halaq, Hannah, Harrison, Hasan, Heather, Holly, Jack, Jacob, Jacqueline, Jake, Jane, Jannine, Jason, Jay, Jeana, Jennifer, Jessica, Jobed, John, Jonathan, Jordan, Joseph, Josh, Judith, Julian, Kate, Kayleigh, Kelsie-Rose, Kieran, Kimberley, Kirsty, Krystyna, Kyle, Laura, Lauren, Leah, Lewis, Logan, Louise, Lucy, Luke, Malcolm, Manuel, Marc, Mark, Martin, Matthew, Michael, Mitchell, Mohammed, Molly, Nadeem, Nathan, Nicola, Nicholas, Olivia, Orazio, Oscar, Owen, Page, Patricia, Peter, Philip, Phillip, Rebecca, Richard, Robert, Ross, Russell, Ryan, Safeen, Samantha, Samuel, Sarah, Scott, Sean, Sebastian, Shahab, Shane, Shaun, Simon, Sophia, Stephen, Stuart, Teresa, Theo, Thomas, Tia, Timothy, William and many others – the real authors of this book

Contents

Introduction: The Long and Winding Road to Tourette Syndrome

Tourette Syndrome: From Witchcraft to Pharmacotherapy

The 'maladie des tics' is currently associated with the name of the French physician who published its first scientific description, Georges Gilles de la Tourette. What is currently known as Tourette syndrome should be more appropriately referred to as 'Gilles de la Tourette syndrome' – after the full surname of the French doctor who published the first comprehensive description of this complex tic disorder. The 1885 article by Gilles de la Tourette featured a case series of nine patients sharing a triad of symptoms encompassing motor/vocal tics (involuntary movements and vocalizations), echolalia (involuntary repetition of others' words) and coprolalia (involuntary swearing). The current definition of Tourette syndrome as a complex chronic tic disorder focuses on the presence of multiple motor tics plus at least one vocal tic, whereas complex vocal tics such as echolalia and coprolalia are not included in the diagnostic criteria. However, this is only the most recent part of a long history that dates back to ancient times. The earliest written record of a possible case of Tourette syndrome might date back to Suetonius' biography of Roman emperor Claudius (in the classical world) and to the description of a priest afflicted with uncontrollable thrusting of his tongue reported in the *Malleus Maleficarum* (in the fifteenth century). It is perhaps not surprising that in the pre-scientific mystic-religious era, tic disorders were seen as a sign of a weak mind or as the effects of supernatural powers – something that could suddenly make otherwise healthy and sound individuals move and shout against their will. At around the same time, one of the first and most elegant descriptions of the involuntary nature of certain abnormal movements (tremor) was produced by Leonardo da Vinci (1452–1519): 'move their trembling parts ... without the permission of the soul'.

Individuals with tics attracted medical attention for the first time in France at the beginning of the nineteenth century. In 1825, Jean Itard (1775–1838), director of the Royal Institute for Deaf Mutes in Paris, published the case of Marquise de Dampierre, a French noblewoman who became famous because of her involuntary movements and obscene utterances. A 1873 monograph by the famous French physician Armand Trousseau described several patients with motor and vocal tics. In 1884, British neurologist John Hughlings-Jackson published a single case report on a patient with tics seen in London. Despite these earlier publications, Georges Gilles de la Tourette (1857–1904) was the first person to characterize the various features of the condition that bears his name, thus pioneering the recognition of Tourette syndrome as a neurological disorder (Figure A). Interestingly, Gilles de la Tourette's landmark 1885 publication included a reappraisal of the

1

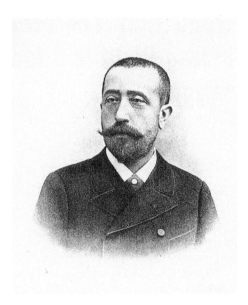

Figure A Georges Gilles de la Tourette (1857–1904).

case of the Marquise de Dampierre and briefly mentioned (in a mildly critical way) Trousseau's observations on the nature of tics. The incorporation of Gilles de la Tourette's name into the eponym was promoted by Gilles de Tourette's mentor, Jean-Martin Charcot (1825–93), who has been deservedly referred to as the father of modern neurology (Figures B and C).

According to Meige and Feindel's influential 1902 study 'Les tics et leur traitement', only a minority of persons with tics fit Gilles de la Tourette's initial description. These authors argued that most tics resulted from uncorrected infantile habits in a population with hereditary weakness. Meige and Feindel's hereditary view proved compatible with eugenics, and it also paved the way to Freudian explanations of early childhood sexual repressive conflict. The first modern clinical-descriptive stage was followed by a psychoanalytic-psychosocial stage: since the French neurologists did not have any definitive explanation for tic disorders other than a sign of degeneration, psychoanalysts postulated a psychological basis. In 1893, Sigmund Freud (1856–1939) wrote that the multiple tic disorder was neurotic in nature and that its cause could only be found by delving into the unconscious. In 1921, Hungarian psychiatrist Sándor Ferenczi (1873–1933) referred to tics as 'stereotyped masturbatory equivalents'. Along these lines, in 1948, Eduard Ascher, professor of psychiatry at the Johns Hopkins University, suggested that the complex tics echolalia and coprolalia were 'related to certain attitudes … toward one or both parents, and also constituted an attempt to suppress their expression'. Under the guidance of psychoanalyst Margaret Mahler (1897–1985), a generation of American psychiatrists learned that the symptoms described by Gilles de la Tourette were signs of a deeper psychosexual disturbance, albeit informed by organic factors. Mahler's clinical case histories led to the

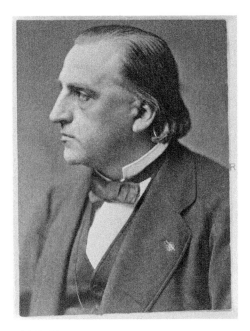

Figure B Jean-Martin Charcot (1825–93).

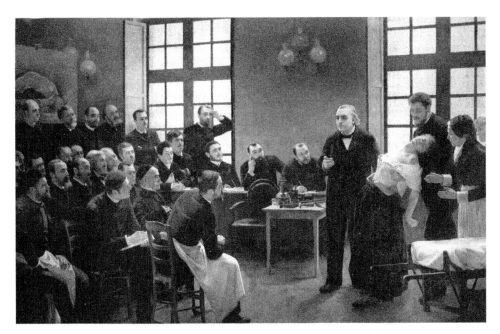

Figure C *Une Leçon Clinique à la Salpêtrière* (A Clinical Lesson at the Salpêtrière), André Brouillet (1887). Charcot is standing next to the patient, and his pupil Gilles de la Tourette is sitting in the front.

conclusion that tic disorders resisted psychoanalytic interventions because the role of the tic was the last 'desperate defense against psychosis'.

Seignot's 1961 scientific report of a case of Tourette syndrome effectively treated with Haloperidol promoted a further 'paradigm shift' from the psychoanalytic theories to the current genetic and neurochemical theories on the aetiology and pathogenesis of Tourette syndrome. Seignot's observation was replicated throughout the world, starting with Caprini and Melotti's case report, which was published in the same year. The introduction of a pharmacological agent to control tics led to the speculation about a neurochemical substrate upon which medications work. Specifically, the unprecedented success of Haloperidol in controlling tics by blocking dopamine receptors in the brain pointed towards a possible excess of dopaminergic neurotransmission. American psychiatrists Arthur and Elaine Shapiro championed the description of Tourette syndrome as a neurological disorder that by definition stood in opposition to psychoanalytic claims. The psychoanalytic perspective was successfully challenged in a book on Tourette syndrome published by the Shapiros in 1978. This paradigm shift in turn kindled interest in tracing the genetic basis of Tourette syndrome, a line of research which has flourished since the 1970s. Throughout the 1980s, studies on other first-generation anti-dopaminergic medications, as well as alpha-2 adrenergic medications, were published, whereas in the 1990s, the second generation of anti-dopaminergic medications were developed. During the first decade of the new millennium, Aripiprazole (sometimes referred to as 'third-generation anti-dopaminergic medication') was first shown to be characterized by good efficacy and tolerability in the treatment of tics. More recently, a range of other medications belonging to different pharmaceutical classes have been investigated in patients with Tourette syndrome. The vast majority of these medications are pharmacological agents initially developed to treat other neuropsychiatric conditions.

In general, the efficiency of medication research and development, measured simply in terms of the number of new drugs brought to market by the global biotechnology and pharmaceutical industries per research and development spending, has declined fairly steadily. This negative trend has been referred to as 'Eroom's Law', in contrast to the more familiar Moore's Law (spelled backwards), the law that describes the exponential increase in the number of transistors that can be placed at a reasonable cost onto an integrated circuit. Figures show that this number doubled every two years from the 1970s to 2010, and the term Moore's Law is now used more generally for technologies that improve exponentially over time. On the contrary, in the US, it has been observed that the number of new Food and Drug Administration–approved medications per billion dollars of research and development spending in the drug industry has halved approximately every 9 years since 1950, in inflation-adjusted terms. The different degree of complexity and limited current understanding of biological systems versus the relative simplicity and higher level of understanding of solid-state physics and information technology explains part of the contrast between Moore's Law and Eroom's Law. It is also possible that Eroom's Law in pharmacology is related to the so-called *better than the Beatles problem* ('imagine how hard it would be to achieve commercial success with new pop songs if any new song had to be better than the Beatles, if the entire Beatles catalogue was available for free, and if people did not get bored with old Beatles records'). It has been suggested that something similar applies to the discovery and development of new medications, and the pharmacotherapy of Tourette syndrome is no exception to this wider trend.

Rational Pharmacotherapy for Tics

In 2014 the Tourette Association of America described Tim Howard, the former goalkeeper of English Premier League football teams and of the US national soccer team, as 'the most notable person in the world with the condition' and conferred on him their Champion of Hope Award. Interestingly, in his autobiography *The Keeper* (2014) and associated media interviews, Howard stated that he does not take or advocate pharmacotherapy, referring to such treatment as 'a concoction of drugs for other ailments' and suggesting that anti-tic medications 'make you drowsy, make you zombie-like'. Indeed, a 2015 systematic review of the prevalence and management of the adverse effects of anti-dopaminergic drugs, the most commonly used medications for tic control, was titled 'First Do No Harm'. It is widely acknowledged that the adverse effects of anti-dopaminergic medications are diverse and common, albeit not often systematically assessed, with a potential negative impact on adherence and engagement. There is some evidence suggesting that parents of young patients with Tourette syndrome have concerns about adverse effects of medications for tics, especially anti-dopaminergic agents. However, there is also evidence that young patients with Tourette syndrome and parents of young patients with Tourette syndrome can have positive perceptions of anti-tic medication. A large UK-based study published in 2015 explored how these two groups of participants perceive different treatment strategies for tics. In addition to the known concerns and limitations about taking medication for tics (mainly regarding the perceived adverse effects and limited beneficial effects), there were interesting reports on the positive experiences of medication for tics. Specifically, young patients with Tourette syndrome who had taken medication for tics felt that it helped them to reduce their tics or to have better control over them. A considerable proportion of participants reported that medication for tics allowed them to feel less self-conscious about their tics and to disguise them better when in public. A few of the participants who endorsed this theme commented specifically on the dopamine receptor partial agonist Aripiprazole: for example, 'I find Aripiprazole helps quite a lot actually-I am not as bad as I was. I don't have many tics during the day or anything anymore'. Parents also identified that medication could be helpful for the children's tics. Another important theme that emerged from this study is the patients' and parents' concern that health care professionals have limited knowledge of Tourette syndrome, with relevant implications in terms of accessing and receiving evidence-based treatment. These findings are in line with the results of a previous study conducted in Spain, in which young patients with Tourette syndrome and their parents described difficulties receiving a diagnosis of Tourette syndrome that were associated with a lack of knowledge regarding tics among health care professionals. Moreover, since pharmacotherapy is a common treatment for tics, young patients and their families may value receiving clear information regarding the rationale for using medications and their potential adverse effects.

In writing this book, it was the author's goal to fill a gap in the rapidly expanding literature on Tourette syndrome by producing a handy reference manual directed at movement disorders specialists and professionals treating patients with tics, but potentially useful to anyone interested in the pharmacological therapy of tics. This book's practical approach and pocket size should make it a particularly valuable resource for medical practitioners working in busy clinics with patients with Tourette syndrome and other tic disorders. The text is divided into three parts. Part I covers background information of practical use to diagnose Tourette syndrome and assess tic severity. Specifically, the first chapter focuses on the clinical evaluation and differential diagnosis of tics and related disorders, whereas the second chapter is devoted to the use of psychometric instruments, encompassing recommended rating scales for tic severity, premonitory urges and quality of life. Part II consists of four chapters on the most widely used pharmacological options for tics, grouped according to their mechanisms of action (first- and second-generation anti-dopaminergic medications, alpha-2 adrenergic medications and other tic-suppressing medications). Within each chapter, individual medications are presented in alphabetical order for easier information gathering, thus enabling physicians to use the text as a stand-alone reference in busy clinical settings, such as specialist movement disorders clinics or general neurology ward rounds. Particular care has been taken in covering the key medications used for tic control, detailing for each agent the main pharmacodynamic and pharmacokinetic properties, relevant medicinal forms, titration schedules, indications, contra-indications, tolerability profiles, clinically relevant interactions and recommendations for use in special populations. This information is followed by a summary of the behavioural neurology profile and the recommendations for the use of each medication according to published guidelines on the treatment of tics. Each monograph closes with a section providing a visual overall rating in terms of efficacy for tics and behavioural problems, as well as tolerability of the medication, again drawing on the existing evidence. While the underlying pharmacology is presented to provide a quick refresher and background on the underlying mechanisms, the text has been deliberately focused to cover practical aspects related to the pharmacotherapy of tics following the most up-to-date evidence-based guidance. However, it is important to note that most recommendations on clinical practice in the field of behavioural neurology are empirical, as data based on methodologically sound research are often lacking. Coherence is maintained by the use of a standard template for each medication, with consistency in both required information and writing style. Finally, the existing international guidelines on the pharmacotherapy of tics (based on systematic literature review/meta-analysis and expert consensus) are described in two chapters within Part III.

In line with the practical aims of the book, particular care has been taken in the selection of the references at the end of the volume: a list of primary sources which could serve as first ports of call for readers who are keen to explore in greater depth the clinically relevant information presented in a concise way within each chapter. The vast majority of the referenced work therefore consists in review articles and books published over the past two decades, with a few notable exceptions (Figure D). The presented material was also selected in an attempt to highlight how the behavioural neurology/neuropsychiatry approach could open up privileged avenues to the understanding of the expression of tics and co-morbid behavioural symptoms in patients with Tourette syndrome.

Most of the text is devoted to the illustration of the pharmacotherapy of tics, with only brief mention of other treatment options, such as neurosurgery (deep brain stimulation), which is a more invasive approach still at a pioneering stage, and behavioural interventions, which are more established interventions and would probably deserve more space or a separate book. This is only one of the several shortcomings of the present work, which will not have escaped the attention of more learned readers. Behavioural neurologists and neuropsychiatrists are probably among the best placed readers to appreciate that accuracy and comprehensiveness have often been sacrificed on the altar of simplification and conciseness. It is to them that the author's most sincere apologies should go, in the hope that

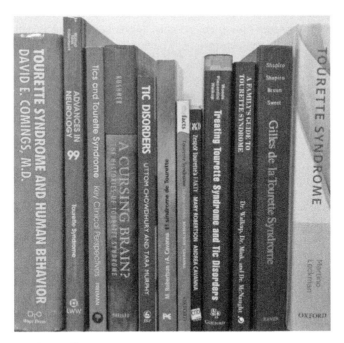

Figure D Tourette syndrome: a library.

these are not sacrifices made in vain. Important omissions encompass the treatment of the behavioural co-morbidities of Tourette syndrome, which can affect health-related quality of life to a higher extent than tics. There is, however, mention of the clinically relevant role of anti-dopaminergic medications for tic-related obsessive-compulsive disorder and alpha-2 adrenergic agonists for co-morbid attention-deficit hyperactivity disorder. Moreover, the list of anti-tic medications is far from exhaustive. For example, there are no chapters on the newer and not-yet-established treatments for tics that are currently under investigation, such as the newer anti-dopaminergic medication Ecopipam and cannabinoids. Finally, the information about medication dosages and indications is based on data from adult populations.

After psychoeducation, the first important step in the management of Tourette syndrome is the optimization of treatment interventions in patients presenting with tics and co-morbid behavioural symptoms. The present book aims to be a pocket-sized guide to assist neurologists in the use of pharmacotherapy when treating patients with Tourette syndrome and associated behavioural problems. Psychiatrists treating patients with neurodevelopmental conditions might also find in this volume a useful tool for their clinical practice. It is expected that the prescribing habits of treating clinicians are based on a better understanding of the nature of tics, the characteristics of the patients and the principles of rational pharmacotherapy. Rational pharmacotherapy processes include choosing suitable medications, at an optimum dose and duration of use, among the effective and safe pharmacological options that are available. Providing patients with accurate information about the diagnosis and treatment is equally important in order to optimize the risk-benefit ratio of the chosen medications. The borderlands between neuropharmacology and psychopharmacology chartered in this book should offer valuable resources to treating clinicians who prioritize health-related quality of life as a therapeutic outcome for their patients. It has been noted that there can be two explanations for the surprisingly low prevalence of persons displaying tics in the street scene: the alleviating effect of medication and the tendency of persons with Tourette syndrome to avoid public spaces. It is the author's hope that this book contributes to make the former explanation more likely than the latter.

Evaluation and Differential Diagnosis of Tics and Related Disorders

Clinical Characteristics of Tics

Tourette syndrome is a neurodevelopmental condition characterized by multiple tics. A tic is a sudden, rapid, repetitive, non-rhythmic movement (e.g. eye blinking) or vocalization (e.g. throat clearing). Tics are often described as semi-voluntary or 'unvoluntary', as, strictly speaking, they are neither voluntary nor involuntary, but may be experienced as a voluntary response to an unwanted distressing sensation called 'premonitory urge'. Premonitory urges are physical 'build-up' sensations to perform specific tics, which are perceived as suppressible yet irresistible, similar to the need to sneeze or scratch an itch. Patients often describe the need to tic as the mounting of inner tension, localized either to the body region where the tic is about to occur or throughout the body. Tic expression is typically associated with a transient sensation of relief.

Tics are arbitrarily classified as being either motor or vocal. Motor tics are associated with movement, while vocal tics are associated with sound and are more appropriately referred to as phonic tics, because the vocal cords are not involved in all tics that produce sound. The division between motor and vocal tics is somewhat artificial, as vocal tics are essentially motor tics involving the nose, mouth, throat and larynx, resulting in the concomitant production of different sounds. Tics can be described based on their anatomical location, number, frequency and duration. Another useful descriptor of tics is their intensity or 'forcefulness', as certain tics call attention to themselves simply by virtue of their exaggerated, forceful character. Motor tics can be simple or complex, according to whether they involve isolated muscles or multiple muscular districts, often in an orchestrated pattern. Likewise, meaningless sounds are referred to as simple vocal tics, whereas words are referred to as complex vocal tics. Complex tics can include echophenomena (echopraxia: copying other people's movements; echolalia: repeating other people's words), paliphenomena (palipraxia: repeating one's own actions; palilalia: repeating one's own words a set number of times or until it feels 'just right') and coprophenomena (copropraxia: rude gestures as tics; coprolalia: swearing as a tic) (Table 1.1). The prevalence of coprolalia – arguably the most widely known manifestation of Tourette syndrome – ranges from 10 per cent (in the community) to 30 per cent (in specialist clinics). Based on the nature and duration of the muscular contraction, tics can also be categorized as clonic (abrupt in onset and rapid), tonic (isometric contraction of the involved body part) or dystonic (sustained abnormal posture).

Individual patients present with their own tic repertoires, constantly changing patterns of motor and vocal tics, with different subsets of tics being present at different life stages, alongside a possible core of more stable tics present since onset. The range of observed tics is extraordinary, so that virtually any voluntary movement or vocalization the human body can produce can emerge as a tic. It is important to take the necessary time to conduct a thorough assessment, as some tics can be invisible to the observer, such as abdominal tensing (Tables 1.2 and 1.3).

Table 1.1 Description of selected complex tics in Tourette syndrome

Coprolalia	Complex vocal tic consisting of involuntary swearing
Copropraxia	Complex motor tic consisting of the involuntary production of obscene gestures
Echolalia	Complex vocal tic consisting of the repetition of other people's words
Echopraxia	Complex motor tic consisting of the imitation of other people's movements
Palilalia	Complex vocal tic consisting of the repetition of one's own words, often for a set number of times or until the words sound 'just right'
Palipraxia	Complex motor tic consisting of the repetition of one's own movements, often for a set number of times or until the movement feels 'just right'

Table 1.2 Most common motor tics

Forehead	Frowning Raising eyebrows
Eyes	Blinking Looking Rolling Staring Winking
Nose	Flaring Smelling Twitching
Mouth	Blowing Breath holding Lip movements Kissing Pouting Opening Pulling to side Smiling Spitting Teeth gnashing Teeth grinding
Tongue	Protrusion Rubbing against teeth Licking
Face	Grimacing Puffing cheeks out Jaw clenching Jaw movements

Table 1.2 (cont.)

Neck and shoulder	Chin on chest/shoulder
	'Hair out of the eyes' flicking
	Head drooping
	Head nodding
	Head turning
	Neck stretching
	Platysma tightening
	Shoulder shrugging
Arms	Bending
	Stretching
Hands	Finger drumming
	Finger flexing
	Fist clenching
	Wrist movements
Torso	Abdominal contractions
	Twisting
Hips	Gluteus squeezing
	Pelvis movements
	Wiggling bottom
Legs	Bending
	Calf tensing
	Kicking
	Knee locking
	Stretching
Feet	Ankle movements
	Toe scratching
Complex motor tics (directed at self/ others/objects)	Abnormal gait
	Adjusting clothes
	Banging
	Bending
	Biting
	Copropraxia
	Echopraxia
	Forced touching
	Hand clapping
	Hair twisting
	Hitting
	Hopping
	Non-obscene socially inappropriate behaviours
	Palipraxia
	Patting

Table 1.2 (cont.)

	Pinching
	Poking
	Pulling
	Putting finger/hand in mouth
	Scratching
	Skipping
	Squatting
	Stamping
	Stroking
	Tapping
	Touching
	Turning

Table 1.3 Most common vocal tics

Simple vocal tics	Animal sounds
	Blowing raspberries
	Burping
	Clicking
	Consonant sounds (e.g. 'sh sh sh', 't t t')
	Coughing
	Fluctuations in pitch
	Gasping
	Growling
	Grunting
	Gulping
	Hiccup
	Hissing
	Hooting
	Moaning
	Noisy breathing
	Panting
	Screaming
	Sniffing
	Snorting
	Squeaking
	Sucking noise
	Throat clearing
	Vocalizations (e.g. ah, ee, eh, ooh, ugh, 'wawa' sounds)
	Wailing
	Whistling
	Yelping

Table 1.3 (cont.)

Complex vocal tics	Coprolalia
	Echolalia
	Isolated words
	Muttering
	Non-obscene socially inappropriate statements
	Palilalia
	Talking to oneself

Table 1.4 Most commonly reported tic-alleviating and tic-exacerbating factors

Tic-alleviating factors	Active concentration
	Distraction from tics
	Music
	Physical exercise
	Relaxation
	Sport
Tic-exacerbating factors	Anxiety
	Boredom
	Excitement
	Exposure to tics (incl. conversation on tics)
	Stress
	Tiredness

Tics are characterized by a spontaneously fluctuating nature ('waxing and waning' course). It has been observed that over the course of hours, tics tend to occur in bouts, with somewhat regular inter-tic intervals. Tics have occasionally been reported to occur during sleep, although most patients become tic-free while asleep. Tics can be voluntarily suppressed for a variable length of time, at the expense of mounting inner tension. Moreover, tic severity may diminish during periods of goal-directed behaviour, when the individual is absorbed in an activity, concentrating, focused or emotionally pleased (mental state of 'flow'). Conversely, tics are typically exacerbated by stress, anxiety, excitement, anger or fatigue. There is inter-individual variability in reported tic-alleviating and tic-exacerbating factors (Table 1.4).

Tics are three to four times more common in males than in females. Once thought to be a rare condition, Tourette syndrome is currently known to be relatively common, with a prevalence of 0.4–1 per cent in school-age children cross-culturally. Milder chronic tic disorders, consisting of either motor or vocal tics (but not both), have a prevalence of approximately 5 per cent, whereas transient tics can be reported at some point by up to 20 per cent of subjects.

Tics typically have their onset between the ages of 4 and 7 years, with the majority manifesting by 10 years. Moreover, by the age of 10 years, most children are aware of the irresistible premonitory urges that precede their tics. The first tics at onset are simple movements, such as eye blinking, nose twitching or facial grimaces; simple motor tics usually progress in a rostro-caudal direction, with a tendency to become more complex over time. Vocal tics typically begin as simple vocalizations, such as throat clearing, sniffing or grunting, after the onset of motor tics, and can also progress from simple vocalizations to more complex ones. In most cases, tics reach their peak in severity between the ages of 10 and 12 years. Although the course of Tourette syndrome is highly variable and difficult to predict, prognosis in early adulthood tends to follow a broad rule of thirds: in one-third of cases, tics virtually completely remit; in one-third, tics improve to a considerable extent; and in one-third, tics persist throughout life, with fluctuating degrees of severity.

The multifaceted clinical characteristics of Tourette syndrome can make it difficult for clinicians to reach a firm diagnosis of the condition. The Tourette Syndrome Diagnostic Confidence Index (DCI) is an instrument developed through a collaborative effort of an expert group of clinicians to assist the diagnostic process of Tourette syndrome (Table 1.5). Based on the range and complexity of tics, their changeable nature, the temporal features of tic expression and associated sensory experiences, the DCI produces a score from 0 to 100 that is a measure of the likelihood of having or ever having had Tourette syndrome. In other words, the DCI is an index to give a confidence level as to whether Tourette syndrome is actually present or was ever present. The mean score among the 280 patients assessed in the DCI validation study was 61 (standard deviation 20).

Diagnostic Criteria of Tic Disorders

Primary tic disorders compose several diagnostic categories within the group of neurodevelopmental disorders (subgroup motor disorders) according to the current edition of the American Psychiatric Association's *Diagnostic and Statistical Manual of Mental Disorders* (DSM-5, published in 2013). These include Tourette syndrome, persistent (chronic) motor or vocal tic disorder, provisional tic disorder and the other specified and unspecified tic disorders. The diagnostic boundaries between different categories are a nosographic convention, as tic disorders are best seen as a continuum (along the 'tic spectrum'): the different tic disorders are likely to represent truncated forms of Tourette syndrome, the fully fledged condition. Specifically, diagnosis for any tic disorder is based on the presence of motor and/ or vocal tics (Criterion A), duration of tic symptoms (Criterion B), age at onset (Criterion C) and absence of any known cause such as another medical condition or substance use (Criterion D). The different tic disorders are hierarchical in order (i.e. Tourette syndrome, followed by persistent motor or vocal tic disorder, followed by provisional tic disorder, followed by the other specified and unspecified tic disorders), such that once a tic disorder at one level of the hierarchy is diagnosed, a lower hierarchy diagnosis cannot be made (Criterion E). Thus, having previously met the diagnostic criteria for Tourette syndrome negates a possible diagnosis of persistent motor or vocal tic disorder. Likewise, a previous diagnosis of persistent motor or vocal tic disorder negates a diagnosis of provisional tic disorder or other specified or unspecified tic disorder. Of note, an additional impairment criterion featured in the DSM-IV (published in 1994); however the set of diagnostic criteria published in the Text Revision edition of the DSM-IV (DSM-IV-TR, 2000) no longer require that tics cause distress or impair functioning.

The current diagnostic criteria of Tourette syndrome are as follows: both multiple motor and one or more vocal tics have been present at some time during the illness, although not necessarily concurrently; the tics may wax and wane in frequency but have persisted for

Table 1.5 Clinical characteristics of Tourette syndrome covered by the Tourette Syndrome Diagnostic Confidence Index, with their weighed scores

Symptom/feature	Weighed score
Coprolalia	15
Complex phonic tics (in addition to simple tics)	12
Complex motor tics (in addition to simple tics)	7
Waxing and waning course of tics	7
Echolalia	5
Echopraxia	5
Palilalia	5
Age at tic onset ≤12 years	4
Orchestrated sequences of tics	4
Premonitory urges to tic	4
Tic variations (appearing/disappearing over time)	4
Tics confirmed by ≥1 reliable observer	4
≥5 motor tic types	2
≥5 phonic tic types	2
Frequent tics (>1/minute at times)	2
Multiple body locations for motor tics	2
Patient sought treatment or diagnosis for tics	2
Tic duration ≥2 years	2
Tic rebound after suppression	2
Tics causing distress	2
Tics suggestible	2
Absence of possible medical causes of tics	1
Attempts to suppress tics	1
First tic over shoulder	1
Relief after tic expression	1
Tics dependent on environmental factors (in addition to stress)	1
Tics voluntarily suppressible	1

more than 1 year since first tic onset; tic onset is before the age of 18 years; and the disturbance is not attributable to the physiological effects of a substance (e.g. cocaine) or another medical condition (e.g. Huntington disease, post-viral encephalitis). The same criteria apply to patients with a diagnosis of 'persistent (chronic) motor or vocal tic disorder', with the exception that single or multiple motor or vocal tics have been present during the illness (but not both motor and vocal tics). Clinicians specify if patients fulfilling

Table 1.6 Key diagnostic features of the main tic disorders (onset before 18 years)

Tic disorder	Number of motor tics	Number of vocal tics	Tics lasting longer than 1 year	Co-morbid ADHD or OCD[a]
Tourette syndrome	2+	1+	yes	very frequent (72%)
Persistent vocal tic disorder	0	1+	yes	frequent (37%)
Persistent motor tic disorder	1+	0	yes	occasional (12%)
Provisional tic disorder[b]	0/1+	0/1+	no	rare (4%)

[a] Community data (school-age children) from Khalifa and Von Knorring (2006). [b]Patients with provisional tic disorder present with at least one motor and/or vocal tic.
Abbreviations: ADHD, attention-deficit hyperactivity disorder; OCD, obsessive-compulsive disorder.

the criteria for this diagnostic category present with motor tics only or with vocal tics only. The diagnostic category of 'provisional tic disorder' is applied to patients who present with single or multiple motor and/or vocal tics that have been present for less than 1 year since first tic onset. As with previous diagnostic categories, tic onset is before the age of 18 years, and the disturbance is not attributable to the physiological effects of a substance or another medical condition. The key diagnostic features of the main tic disorders are summarized in Table 1.6.

The DSM-5 includes two additional categories of tic disorders: other specified and unspecified tic disorders. For other specified or unspecified tic disorders, the movement disorder symptoms are best characterized as tics, but are atypical in presentation or age at onset. There is no duration specification for other specified and unspecified tic disorders. The 'other specified tic disorder' category applies to presentations in which symptoms characteristic of a tic disorder that cause clinically significant distress or functional impairment predominate, but do not meet the full criteria for a tic disorder diagnostic class. The other specified tic disorder category can be followed by the specific reason or failing to meet the criteria for a tic disorder (for example, onset after the age of 18 years). The 'unspecified tic disorder' category is used in situations in which the clinician does not specify the reason for failing to meet the criteria for a tic disorder (for example, presentations in which there is insufficient information to reach a more specific diagnosis).

Differential Diagnosis of Tics and Co-morbid Conditions

The causes of Tourette syndrome and other primary tic disorders are not yet fully understood. Both genetic and non-genetic (environmental) factors have been implicated in the aetiology of Tourette syndrome. Converging findings from both twin and family studies have shown that Tourette syndrome is one of the most heritable, non-Mendelian neurodevelopmental disorders. Tics and/or tic-related symptoms can be traced in family members in the vast majority of cases, although it is known that the clinical manifestations can skip generations. At present genetic tests are not useful in confirming the diagnosis of Tourette syndrome: the extreme variability of the phenotypic expression means that no single gene responsible for the occurrence of tics and Tourette syndrome is considered to be a genetically heterogeneous condition. Non-genetic factors, including pre- and perinatal difficulties as well as post-infectious autoimmunity, have been proposed as possible contributors to the aetiological framework of Tourette syndrome. The hypothesis that Tourette syndrome could belong to a group of conditions called 'paediatric autoimmune neuropsychiatric disorders associated with streptococcal infections' (PANDAS) is still being investigated, although recent findings have led to questioning the possible aetiological role of autoimmune mechanisms. As in most neuropsychiatric disorders, it seems likely that the effects of environmental factors become manifest in genetically predisposed individuals ('the genes load the gun and the environment pulls the trigger').

In addition to Tourette syndrome and other primary tic disorders, a variety of clinical conditions can cause tics. In these cases, the tics are considered secondary to another condition (Table 1.7). Secondary tic disorders are remarkably less common than primary tic disorders and are often evident by the presence of other neurological dysfunction in addition to tics. Therefore diagnostic assessments for secondary causes of tics in the form of neuroimaging investigations or specific blood tests are generally not necessary when confronted with a young patient who has tics in the absence of any other significant neurological deficits.

Probably the most common causes of secondary tics are other neurodevelopmental disorders, especially autism spectrum disorders with or without severe learning disabilities. In pervasive developmental disorders, tics are often accompanied by stereotypies,

Table 1.7 Main causes of secondary tic disorders

Neurodevelopmental disorders	Autism spectrum disorders
	Chromosomal abnormalities
	Developmental stuttering
Neurodegenerative diseases	Huntington disease
	Neurodegeneration with brain iron accumulation
Acquired brain injury	Infections
	Stroke
	Traumatic brain injury
Post-infectious conditions	Post-encephalitis
	Sydenham's chorea
Genetic systemic illnesses	Neuroacanthocytosis
	Wilson disease
Medications	Anti-dopaminergic medications (tardive dyskinesias)
	Anti-epileptic medications
	Central nervous system stimulants
	Levodopa
Toxins	Carbon monoxide
	Mercury
Psychogenic movement disorders	

resulting in challenging presentations in terms of differential diagnosis. Tics have also been observed in patients with developmental stuttering. A number of other genetic developmental disorders (including rare chromosomal abnormalities) affecting the brain have also been reported to be potentially associated with tics.

Tics may accompany other neuropsychiatric symptoms in a few neurodegenerative conditions of genetic origin. Huntington disease is an autosomal dominant disease caused by expanded CAG repeats in the gene for huntingtin on chromosome 4. Since the discovery of the gene, Huntington disease is easily diagnosed by molecular genetic methods. The clinical picture is characterized by choreiform (dance-like) involuntary movements and progressive dementia. Tics have been observed as potential manifestations of the motor presentation of Huntington disease. Neurodegeneration with brain iron accumulation is a rare autosomal recessive disorder linked to mutations of the PANK-2 gene, which codes for the enzyme pantothenate kinase. Clinical symptoms typically present in the second or third decade, with motor manifestations (rigidity, spasticity, and dystonia) and progressive dementia. A few cases with tics have been described in association with this condition.

Acquired brain damage can result in the development of movement disorders. Specifically, tics can rarely occur following brain insults that are either generalized or more focal (usually affecting fronto-striatal pathways connecting the cerebral cortex and the basal ganglia). In addition to rare cases of sudden-onset tics following stroke or traumatic brain injury (mainly resulting in basal ganglia damage), a few post-encephalitic cases of tics have been reported (e.g. herpes encephalitis, varicella zoster encephalitis) in patients with neuroimaging changes within the striatum and midbrain. Secondary motor and vocal tics have been reported to be associated with other central nervous system infections, including HIV, encephalitis, and neuroborreliosis (Lyme disease). It has been recognized that both tics and obsessive-compulsive symptoms can occur as motor and psychiatric manifestations of Sydenham's chorea, previously known as acute rheumatic fever.

Secondary tics have occasionally been reported in rare systemic illnesses of genetic origin. Neuroacanthocytosis is an autosomal recessive illness caused by the presence of abnormal erythrocytes in the blood (acanthocytes). Patients have variable clinical manifestations, which include chorea, parkinsonism, peripheral neuropathy, seizures, as well as lip and tongue biting. Occasionally, patients have been reported to experience tics secondary to neuroacanthocytosis, alongside tic-related obsessive-compulsive symptoms. Wilson disease is a rare metabolic disorder characterized by an autosomal recessive heritability pattern. The pathological process results in accumulation of copper within the brain (basal ganglia), liver and other vital organs. Most patients with Wilson disease are diagnosed between the ages of 5 and 35, when they can present with gastrointestinal symptoms, jaundice, eye discoloration (so-called Kayser–Fleischer rings) and/or involuntary movements that can resemble dystonic tics.

Like other hyperkinetic movement disorders, tics can be the long-lasting manifestation of pharmacologically induced tardive dyskinesias (tardive tics), which occurs following exposure to anti-dopaminergic medications, such as anti-psychotic and anti-emetic agents. Several medications have been reported to temporarily induce tics, including central nervous system stimulants (Methylphenidate, amphetamines, cocaine, heroin), anti-epileptic medications (especially Lamotrigine) and Levodopa. Certain stimulants are used as pharmacotherapy rather than as recreational drugs: specifically, randomized controlled trials have shown that Methylphenidate gradually titrated at the lowest efficacious dose does not exacerbate tics in young patients with Tourette syndrome and is effective in treating co-morbid attention-deficit and hyperactivity disorder. Exposure to certain environmental toxins, including carbon monoxide and mercury, has also been reported as a rare cause of tics.

Finally, tics can be a manifestation of a psychogenic movement disorder (psychogenic tics). Patients with psychogenic tics can have exaggerated or dramatic manifestations, in the absence of simple motor and vocal tics. Other potentially helpful clinical features in establishing a psychogenic aetiology include inconsistencies with the typical presentations of tics, accentuation with suggestion and abnormal reduction with distraction, absence of premonitory sensations, presence of other functional symptoms, associated personality features, inappropriate affect, and underlying psychological conflicts and/or secondary gain.

Due to their heterogeneous clinical phenomenology, the diagnosis of tics can be challenging and requires an in-depth assessment by an experienced clinician, who is able to distinguish tics from other types of motor manifestations (Table 1.8).

Table 1.8 Other motor manifestations resembling tics.

Normal movements	Habits
Movement disorders associated with neurological conditions	Athetosis
	Chorea
	Dystonia
	Myoclonus
	Tremor
Movement disorders associated with psychiatric conditions	Compulsions
	Hyperactivity
	Mannerisms
	Stereotypies

Specifically, tics need to be distinguished from physiological habits, as well as other hyperkinetic movement disorders of neurological origin and movement disorders associated with psychiatric conditions. Habits are normal movements frequently seen in healthy individuals, particularly during times of boredom, anxiety or self-consciousness. Common habits include repetitive, coordinated movements such as finger drumming, foot tapping and hair twirling. Thumb sucking is an example of a developmental habit. Habits are easier to suppress (at least temporarily) than tics and are not preceded by premonitory urges. The presence of premonitory urges appears to be a feature of tics that is not shared by other hyperkinetic movement disorders of neurological origin. Moreover, the co-occurrence of vocal tics can allow the proper identification of body jerks as motor tics. Both myoclonus (lightning-like muscle jerks) and chorea (dance-like muscle jerks) can resemble the sudden twitches of simple motor tics; however, these motor manifestations tend not to be repetitive in the same location like tics. Dystonic tics can resemble the slow, twisting movements and postures of dystonia. Contrary to dystonia, dystonic tics are not continuous, but tend to occur in brief bursts, thus producing abnormal postures that are not as sustained. Tremor is by definition characterized by its rhythmic pattern (high frequency and low amplitude in essential tremor, low frequency and high amplitude in Parkinson disease) and is completely involuntary. Athetosis consists in continuous writhing movements of the hands and feet that are slower than tics and are typically associated with chorea (choreo-athetosis).

Table 1.9 Most common psychiatric and neurological co-morbidities of Tourette syndrome

Psychiatric co-morbidities	ADHD
	Affective disorders
	Anxiety
	ASD
	Impulse control disorders (disruptive behaviour disorders)
	Obsessive-compulsive behaviours/OCD
	Personality disorders
Neurological co-morbidities	Headache
	Sleep disorders

Abbreviations: ADHD, attention-deficit hyperactivity disorder; ASD, autism spectrum disorder; OCD, obsessive-compulsive disorder.

Although tics are the defining aspect of Tourette syndrome, they rarely occur in isolation, and for most patients the co-occurring conditions are the main determinant of health-related quality of life. Tourette syndrome has been referred to as the quintessential neuropsychiatric disorder because of the co-existence of both neurological and psychiatric manifestations. Of note, Tourette syndrome and other tic disorders are included in the classification of both psychiatric disorders (Diagnostic and Statistical Manual of Mental Disorders of the American Psychiatric Association) and neurological disorders (hyperkinetic movement disorders of the Movement Disorder Society). In addition to frequent co-morbid neurological conditions (e.g. headache, sleep disorders), it has been estimated that about 90 per cent of patients with Tourette syndrome present with associated behavioural symptoms. The most commonly reported psychiatric co-morbidities are obsessive-compulsive disorder, attention-deficit and hyperactivity disorder, anxiety, affective disorders, impulse control disorders (characterized by disruptive behaviours), autism spectrum disorders and personality disorders (Table 1.9).

The phenotypic heterogeneity in Tourette syndrome appears to be related to the complex genetic relationships among the tic disorder and the associated behavioural symptoms. The characterization of Tourette syndrome phenotypes based on patterns of co-occurrence of tics and behavioural symptoms is a fundamental prerequisite for the establishment of more precise phenotype-genotype correlations. Large clinical studies using principal component factor analysis, hierarchical cluster analysis and other statistical techniques have started to dissect the clinical spectrum of Tourette syndrome into individual phenotypes. Based on the different degrees of complexity and care needs, patients with Tourette syndrome have been classified into three subgroups: 'pure' Tourette syndrome (patients mainly presenting with simple motor and vocal tics), 'full-blown' Tourette syndrome (patients with both simple and complex tics, such as copro/echo/paliphenomena) and Tourette syndrome 'plus' (patients diagnosed with co-morbid psychiatric disorders) (Table 1.10). Moreover, the high prevalence of behavioural symptoms in patients with Tourette syndrome can pose significant challenges in the differential diagnosis between tics and movement disorders linked to co-morbid psychiatric conditions.

The prevalence of co-morbid obsessive-compulsive disorder in patients with Tourette syndrome ranges from 11 to 66 per cent, although it has been estimated that the prevalence of sub-threshold obsessive-compulsive behaviours could be considerably

Table 1.10 Types of Tourette syndrome

'Pure' Tourette syndrome	Mainly simple motor and vocal tics
'Full-blown' Tourette syndrome	Both simple and complex tics
Tourette syndrome 'plus'	Tourette syndrome with co-morbid psychiatric diagnoses

higher. Compulsions and complex motor tics are sometimes difficult to distinguish, particularly when the two phenomena coexist. In contrast to tics, compulsions are ritualistic, goal-directed behaviours driven by obsessional thoughts (anxiety-generating cognitions). Consistent findings from clinical studies have shown that patients with Tourette syndrome tend to report specific obsessive-compulsive symptoms, that are phenomenologically different from the symptoms reported by patients who have obsessive-compulsive disorder but not tics. Specifically, patients with Tourette syndrome report a significantly higher prevalence of concerns for symmetry, evening-up behaviours, obsessional counting (arithmomania), ordering and 'just right' perceptions, whereas patients with pure forms of obsessive-compulsive disorder have a higher rate of concerns for contamination, as well as cleaning and washing rituals. Examples of tic-related obsessive-compulsive symptoms include repetitive tapping or touching (usually for a set number of times or until it feels 'just right') and have been referred to as 'compulsive tics' or 'compultics'. Tic-related obsessive-compulsive disorder has been proposed as a specific subtype of obsessive-compulsive disorder in patients who have a current or past history of a tic disorder. There appears to be a complex genetic relationship between Tourette syndrome and tic-related obsessive-compulsive disorder, which is also suggested by a high degree of heritability of both conditions. Male preponderance and earlier age at onset compared to obsessive-compulsive disorder without tics are further clinical features which indicate that tic-related obsessive-compulsive disorder could be intrinsic to Tourette syndrome. Moreover, phenomenological differences between tic-related obsessive-compulsive disorder and obsessive-compulsive disorder are likely to reflect different pathophysiological mechanisms and have implications for both the diagnosis and the clinical management of complex cases.

The prevalence of co-morbid attention-deficit and hyperactivity disorder in young patients with Tourette syndrome ranges from 38 per cent (in community settings) to over 60 per cent (in specialist clinics). Behavioural symptoms can present prior to the onset of tics, with three main clinical phenotypes (inattentive, hyperactive-impulsive and combined). Although the severity of attention-deficit and hyperactivity disorder is known to decrease over time, its persistence through key developmental stages can have far-reaching consequences, in particular when academic performance and/or social functioning are affected. Motor tics are fragments of normal movements circumscribed to functional muscle groups, whereas motor symptoms in attention-deficit and hyperactivity disorder consist in general motor hyperactivity. The time course is different: tics occur suddenly and are uniformly repeated (often in bouts), whereas hyperactivity increases slowly and is temporally irregular and intermittent. Certain motor tics characterized by impulsiveness, aggressiveness and social inappropriateness (e.g. punching self or others, or touching a hot stove) are sometimes referred to as 'impulsive tics' or 'impultics'.

Stereotypies are coordinated, rhythmic, repetitive and patterned movements that often occur in patients with autism spectrum disorder. The differences between motor stereotypies and tics can be subtle. Stereotypies occur repeatedly for longer periods of time than tics. With regard to body location, stereotypies frequently involve the hands (e.g. hand flapping) or the entire body (e.g. body rocking) rather than the more common tic locations of the eyes, face, head and shoulders. Stereotypies tend to have an earlier age of onset than tics. Moreover, stereotypies are more difficult to suppress than tics, are not associated with premonitory urges and do not respond to treatment interventions. Finally, mannerisms are unusual characteristic ways of performing normal activities. These include things like an odd gait, a peculiar speech or exaggerated movements that attract attention to an individual. Like stereotypic movements and motor automatisms, mannerisms can be associated with schizophrenia.

Pathophysiology of Tics and Treatment Approaches

The specialist evaluation of patients with tics includes assessment of the most debilitating complaints, ascertains how the symptoms developed and inquires about potential stressors and triggers (Table 1.11).

Table 1.11 Domains of history taking in Tourette syndrome

Demographic data	Age
	Gender
	Ethnicity
	Marital status
	Accommodation
	Education level
	Job status
Tic history	Age at tic onset (first tic at onset)
	Onset after specific illness (throat/chest infections)
	Previous diagnosis of TS (age)
	Course of tic severity (waxing and waning)
	Tic repertoire (lifetime + current tics)
	Premonitory urges
	Tic suppressibility
	Tic-alleviating factors
	Tic-exacerbating factors
Developmental history	Perinatal problems (special care baby unit)
	Developmental delay (milestones)
	Stuttering (speech and language therapy)
	Learning disability (special school)
Family history	Family history of tics
	Family history of TS
	Family history of OCD
	Family history of ADHD
	Family history of other neuropsychiatric conditions

Table 1.11 (cont.)

OCD	Checking
	Counting
	Evening-up/symmetry
	'Just right'
	Obsessional thoughts
ADHD	Inattention
	Hyperactivity
	Impulsivity
Anxiety and affective symptoms	Anxiety
	Depression
	Mood swings
Disruptive behaviours	Anger control problems
	Aggression to people
	Aggression to property
	Self-injurious behaviours
Addictions	Smoking
	Alcohol abuse
	Recreational drugs
	Other addictions
Physical health	Pain symptoms
	Sleep problems
	Allergies
	Other medical problems
Treatment	Current medications (duration, dose, effectiveness, tolerability)
	Previous medications (duration, dose, effectiveness, tolerability, reason for discontinuation)
	Other treatments
	Other previous treatments

Abbreviations: ADHD, attention-deficit hyperactivity disorder; OCD, obsessive-compulsive disorder; TS, Tourette syndrome.

Specifically, both age at onset of the first tic and tic course are recorded. Moreover, information is obtained about which tics are considered to be most distressing by the patients, and about their physical consequences (including pain/injury of muscles and joints). Somatosensory phenomena (premonitory urges) accompanying the tics, tic suppressibility and tic-alleviating and exacerbating factors are covered. The clinical examination of tics is accompanied by a standardized assessment of co-morbid conditions, encompassing obsessive-compulsive behaviours, attention-deficit and hyperactivity symptoms, anxiety, affective symptoms, impulsivity, sleep problems, headache and other medical problems. Collection of the family history should be focused on the presence of tics, obsessive-compulsive behaviours and symptoms of attention-deficit and hyperactivity disorder in close family members. During the clinical interview, a thorough developmental history is obtained. Patients are also asked about family functioning, social network, education/job, financial and housing situation. If available, hetero-anamnesis on tic and disease status can be obtained from a partner, relative or close friend of the patient. An accurate and comprehensive collection of clinical information forms the basis of one of the most important processes in the management of patients with Tourette syndrome: diagnosis communication and psychoeducation should be tailored to the clinical presentation and characteristics of the individual patient.

The diagnosis of tics remains a clinical one, and is based on the historical report and direct observation of motor and vocal manifestations consistent with the phenomenology of tics. Confirming the presence of tics and ascertaining a family history of tics require agreement between clinicians and patients around the definition of tics: sharing this information represents the first pillar of the educational intervention for tic disorders. Appropriate education of patients and their families should cover the phenomenology, natural history, impact on social, academic and professional functioning, relation to environmental factors, behavioural co-morbidities and therapeutic options (Table 1.12). The administration of validated rating scales for tics and premonitory urges is advisable for a correct management approach.

It has been observed that simply providing a diagnostic label is insufficient to prevent misconceptions, negative attitudes and stigma. Psychoeducation is the cornerstone of treatment in patients with primary tic disorders. In fact, it is a crucial step in facilitating a better understanding of the nature of the disorder and it is often the only necessary treatment intervention. Trough appropriate psychoeducation, it is possible to ultimately increase symptom awareness and acceptance for patients and their families. Major educational challenges include dissecting the complex phenomena of 'unvoluntariness' of tics and voluntary 'suppressibility', which may often lead to an excessively blaming attitude of family/partner towards the patient, and may enhance tic-related stress in the family life. The same applies to teachers and colleagues in the school and work environment, respectively. In these environments discrimination and victimization are sources of stigma across

Table 1.12 Key elements of diagnosis communication and psychoeducation in Tourette syndrome

Main features of tics and premonitory urges (including 'unvoluntariness', suppressibility, tic-modulating factors, natural course of tics, tic-related behavioural problems)

Causes, brain mechanisms and available therapeutic options for tics

Effects of different emotional reactions to tics (risk of excessive emotional charge of discussions around tics)

Impact of tics on personal, social, academic or professional activities

Focus on the individual's strengths and interests in supporting efforts to better manage tics and related disorders

Awareness of the dynamics of stigma and discriminating attitudes towards tics

Relevance of sharing adequate information with peers, teachers and/or colleagues

Opportunity of promoting a psychoeducational intervention towards teachers, school friends, employers and/or colleagues to prevent stigma and discrimination in school and work environments different age groups and should be the object of targeted interventions both at an individual level and via outreach measures. It has also been noted that parents' emotional responses to tics may lead to excessive emotional charge of family scenarios, potentially enhancing tics and generating a vicious cycle fuelled by psychosocial stress. A 'matter-of-fact' attitude, thus neither hostile nor excessively accommodating, has been advocated as a useful approach in the family environment. For example, non-derogatory use of humour to deflate emotionally charged interactions can be helpful. Another important area of psychoeducation is the joint evaluation, together with patients and families, of the impact of tics on the ability to fulfil patients' aspirations and express their full potential in the different areas of functioning. Measures used to enhance self-esteem, such as encouraging independence, strong friendships and the exploration of interests, are crucial to ensuring positive adulthood outcome. Finally, psychoeducation should protect both patients and their families from inaccurate information available on the Internet, similar to what is observed with several other medical conditions.

The complexity of the heterogeneous presentations of Tourette syndrome suggests an equally complex pathophysiology. Specifically, multiple pathophysiological mechanisms might be responsible for the expression of different clinical phenotypes. At least three parallel cortico-striato-thalamo-cortical circuits, linking specific cortical regions to subcortical nuclei (basal ganglia and thalamus), are thought to be involved in the pathophysiology of Tourette syndrome: the habitual behavioural circuit, the goal-directed circuit and the emotion-related limbic circuit. The latter circuit might play a key role in the behavioural and emotional aspects of Tourette syndrome, as it connects the basal ganglia with the limbic system via inputs from the hippocampus, amygdala, prefrontal cortex and anterior cingulate gyrus to the ventral striatum (also called nucleus accumbens) (Figure 1.1). The different components of the basal ganglia (sensorimotor, associative and limbic pathways) can explain the co-occurrence of motor and non-motor symptoms in Tourette syndrome.

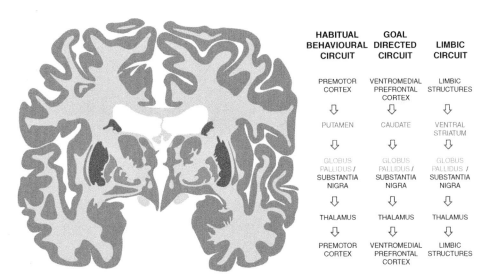

Figure 1.1 Basal ganglia circuitries possibly involved in the pathophysiology of Tourette syndrome.

Both excitatory and inhibitory pathways at the level of cortico-basal ganglia networks have been shown to be involved in the pathophysiology of Tourette syndrome. Alterations in dopaminergic neurotransmission appear to be primarily implicated, although research findings have also highlighted abnormalities within other neurochemical systems (serotonin, glutamate, acetylcholine), as well as inhibitory GABAergic pathways and dopamine-modulating histaminergic neurotransmission. The differential involvement of neural networks and neurochemical systems associated with the pathophysiology of tics and behavioural symptoms is likely to explain at least in part the phenotypical heterogeneity of Tourette syndrome. It is therefore useful to highlight that available pharmacological agents that have been found to suppress tics exert multiple actions at the level of different neurochemical systems. This is particularly relevant to anti-dopaminergic medications, as the most commonly prescribed class of medications for tics and associated behavioural symptoms exert their pharmacological effects at the level of multiple receptor subtypes (Table 1.13). Finally, it has been suggested that the processes of tic generation, tic expression and tic suppression might be associated with the activity of different brain networks. For example, the results of functional neuroimaging studies have shown activation patterns within extra-motor areas (including insula and cingulate cortex) concomitant to premonitory urges, suggesting their possible involvement in tic generation.

The currently incomplete understanding of the pathophysiology of Tourette syndrome has implications for the rational approach to pharmacotherapy: this needs to be bespoke to meet the individual needs suggested by the clinical presentation and personal history of each

Table 1.13 Pharmacological effects of anti-dopaminergic medications on the main receptor subtypes

Action on receptor	Effect(s)
D2 antagonism/partial agonism	Anti-psychosis (positive symptoms), anti-mania, EPS, hyperprolactinaemia (not with partial agonism)
H1 antagonism	Sedation, anti-anxiety, weight gain, anti-nausea
M1 antagonism	Sedation, anti-anxiety, dry mouth, blurred vision, constipation, urinary retention, sinus tachycardia, cognitive problems, anti-EPS
Alpha-1 antagonism	Sedation, anti-anxiety, postural hypotension, dizziness
Alpha-2 antagonism	Anti-depression, improved cognition
5-HT1A antagonism/partial agonism	Anti-depression, anti-anxiety, anti-mania, improved cognition, anti-EPS
5-HT1B antagonism	Anti-depression
5-HT1D antagonism	Anti-depression
5-HT2A antagonism	Sedation, anti-mania, anti-EPS, improved cognition
5-HT2C antagonism	Anti-depression, improved cognition, weight gain
5-HT3 antagonism	Anti-depression
5-HT7 antagonism	Anti-depression, anti-anxiety, improved cognition

Abbreviations: 5-HT, serotonergic; Alpha, adrenergic; D, dopaminergic; EPS, extrapyramidal symptoms; H, histaminergic; M, muscarinic (cholinergic).

patient. Active interventions for tics are usually considered when tics cause physical and/or psychosocial impairment. However there is a high degree of inter-individual variability in both when and how tics can cause impairment, affect patients' quality of life and diminish their life achievements. In addition to interference with daily life activities, frequent motor and vocal tics may cause pain or discomfort from repetitive muscle activation or joint motion and interfere with concentration on tasks. Loud vocal tics may attract unwanted attention and disrupt social life, to the point that some patients may avoid social interactions altogether because of fear of embarrassment. The decision to pursue active interventions and commence pharmacotherapy should be a collaborative one between patient and clinician, with the patient deciding if medications are necessary and the clinician providing expertise on which agents should be considered, at which dose and in which order. Prior to starting any medication, it is important to provide patients with counselling on treatment expectations, since pharmacotherapy (like any other treatment intervention for tics) rarely abolishes tics entirely, but can provide meaningful reduction in both tic frequency and severity. Finally, in consideration of the fluctuating course of tics and the natural history of tic disorders, it can be appropriate to periodically taper and discontinue medications to determine if they are still necessary. The identification of predictors and moderators of response to the different pharmacological classes, as well as the definition of refractoriness to pharmacological treatment for tics, are still among the many open questions in this field.

Chapter 2

Assessment of Tic Severity

The assessment and quantification of tics can pose considerable difficulties because of a number of factors, including the spontaneous fluctuations of tic severity and the tendency of patients to suppress their tics, especially when in the consultation room with the clinician. It is therefore advisable to supplement direct observation and clinical interviewing (including historical and external information whenever available) with the use of psychometric instruments validated in patients with Tourette syndrome. Information can be obtained from patients or from informants such as parents and teachers, through questionnaire constructs. For Tourette syndrome, most available instruments are parent- and/or teacher-rated questionnaires in childhood and self-report scales in adolescence and adulthood (Table 2.1).

In addition to quantifying clinically relevant phenomena in patients with tics, the use of standardized rating scales in routine clinical practice allows the monitoring of the course of tics and behavioural symptoms. This is particularly relevant to clinical research studies on treatment interventions, which have the potential to inform optimal patient care. In order for data to be accurate and of clinical utility, clinical rating scales need to have adequate psychometric properties, including reliability and validity. Good reliability is an indication that the scale produces the same information when individuals are tested by the same raters at different times (test-retest reliability), and when the same individual is assessed by different raters (inter-rater reliability). Validity represents a measure of how accurately the instrument captures the theoretical construct of what it aims to assess.

A systematic review of the psychometric properties and use of severity rating and screening instruments for tics and associated sensory phenomena was conducted by an ad hoc subcommittee of the Committee on Rating Scale Development of the International Parkinson's Disease and Movement Disorder Society. The final report, published in 2017, provides clinicians and researchers with helpful guidance on scale selection. The subcommittee adopted the terminology and criteria of the International Parkinson's and Movement Disorders Society Committee on Rating Scales Development: each psychometric instrument was rated as 'recommended' if it had been applied to tic disorders populations, there had been studies on its use beyond the group that developed the scale, and it had been found sufficiently valid, reliable and responsive to change; 'suggested' if it had been applied to tic disorders populations, but only one of the other criteria applied; 'listed' if the instrument had been applied to tic disorders populations, but did not meet other criteria. The choice of the psychometric instruments for use in patients with Tourette syndrome is based on several contextual factors (related to the characteristics of the patient and the clinical context), in addition to the psychometric properties of the individual rating scales (Table 2.2).

Table 2.1 Recommended rating scales for patients with Tourette syndrome

Scales for different symptoms	Respondent	Administration time (minutes)
Tics and associated symptoms		
Motor Tic, Obsessions and Compulsions, Vocal Tic Evaluation Survey (MOVES)	Clinician-rated (recommended for screening); patient-rated (suggested)	5
Shapiro Tourette Syndrome Severity Scale (STSSS)	Clinician-rated (recommended)	5
Tourette's Disorder Scale (TODS)	Clinician-rated (recommended); parent-rated (recommended)	20
Tourette Syndrome–Clinical Global Impression (TS-CGI)	Clinician-rated (recommended)	2
Yale Global Tic Severity Scale (YGTSS)	Clinician-rated (recommended)	20
Premonitory urges		
Premonitory Urge for Tics Scale (PUTS)	Patient-rated (>10 years) (recommended)	5
Individualized Premonitory Urge for Tics Scale (I-PUTS)	Clinician-rated	Variable
Quality of life		
Gilles de la Tourette Syndrome–Quality of Life Scale (GTS-QOL)	Patient-rated	15
Gilles de la Tourette Syndrome–Quality of Life Scale in children and adolescents (C&A-GTS-QOL)	Clinician-rated (6–12 years); patient-rated (13–18 years)	15

Rating Scales for Tic Severity

Motor Tic, Obsessions and Compulsions, Vocal Tic Evaluation Survey (MOVES)

The Motor Tic, Obsessions, Vocal Tic Evaluation Survey (MOVES) is a self-report assessment of the intrinsic symptoms of Tourette syndrome: motor and vocal tics, tic-associated phenomena (complex tics such as echophenomena and coprophenomena), obsessions and compulsions. In addition to yielding total scores, individual scores from the 20 items can be combined in groups of four to produce sub-scores on five sub-scales: motor tics, vocal tics, associated symptoms, obsessions and compulsions. Patients are asked to rate the frequency of their symptoms over the previous 4 weeks, on a 4-point scale ('never', 'sometimes', 'often', 'always'). The MOVES is a relatively straightforward instrument, brief and easy to administer and to score (up to 5 minutes). A number of psychometric properties were tested and

Table 2.2 Proposed psychometric battery for tics (rating scales of choice) in specialist clinics

Clinical variable	Recommended scale	Rationale
Tics (clinician-rated)	Yale Global Tic Severity Scale (YGTSS)[a]	The most extensively validated and widely used tic-rating instrument; allows the comprehensive, reliable and valid assessment of tic severity across multiple dimensions
Tics (patient-rated)	Motor Tic, Obsessions and Compulsions, Vocal Tic Evaluation Survey (MOVES)	Brief self-report scale that allows assessment of the frequency of tics, associated phenomena, obsessions and compulsions
Premonitory urges (patient-rated)	Premonitory Urge for Tics Scale (PUTS)	Brief self-report scale that allows assessment of the frequency of premonitory urges; extensive psychometric testing carried out
Premonitory urges (clinician-rated)	Individualized Premonitory Urge for Tics Scale (I-PUTS)	Reliable and valid measure capturing multiple dimensions (number, frequency, intensity and body region location) of premonitory urges
Quality of life (patient-rated)	Gilles de la Tourette Syndrome–Quality of Life Scale (GTS-QOL) and Gilles de la Tourette Syndrome–Quality of Life Scale in children and adolescents (C&A-GTS-QOL)	Disease-specific instruments for the assessment of quality of life across the lifespan

[a] The relatively long administration time of the YGTSS could be a hindrance to its routine use in busy clinical settings. Two other recommended rating scales, the Shapiro Tourette Syndrome Severity Scale (STSSS) and the Tourette Syndrome–Clinical Global Impression (TS-CGI), can be used as alternative options, especially when it is not necessary to capture all dimensions of tic severity and a more rapid rating is preferable.

proved satisfactory. The validity of the MOVES was demonstrated by its strong correlations to two clinician-rated measures of tic severity and obsessive-compulsive symptom severity, with evidence of sensitivity to clinically relevant changes. Specifically, convergent validity was acceptable across all ages, as shown by the correlation coefficients for the MOVES tics sub-scale – compared to the YGTSS total tic severity score: 0.7 ($p<0.001$); compared to the Tourette Syndrome Global Scale (TSGS): 0.73 ($p<0.001$). With regard to reliability, a few sub-scales of the MOVES showed below standard (<0.70) correlation coefficients: tics (0.54), associated symptoms (0.40), total scores (0.69). Nevertheless, the MOVES is widely recognized as a useful measure of patient perception on tic symptoms, in order to complement clinician ratings in the protocols of descriptive and/or treatment studies. The French version of the MOVES showed equally good psychometric properties: the cross-cultural adaptation of this instrument allows clinicians to assess French-speaking patients with Tourette syndrome aged 12 years and over. Despite having been designed as a self-report severity scale, the MOVES has also been tested as a comprehensive screening instrument for tics and tic-related behavioural symptoms. A cut-off score of 10 showed the best diagnostic performance versus psychiatric diagnostic criteria (DSM-III-R criteria), with adequate sensitivity (87 per cent), specificity (94 per cent), positive and negative predictive values (90 per cent and 94 per cent, respectively). In 2017, the report of the Committee on Rating Scale Development of the Movement Disorders Society rated the MOVES as a 'recommended' clinician-rated screening instrument and as a 'suggested' patient-rated tic severity measure. The MOVES did not reach a higher level of recommendation as tic severity measure because of the lack of data on its divergent validity, internal consistency and responsiveness.

Shapiro Tourette Syndrome Severity Scale (STSSS)

The Shapiro Tourette Syndrome Severity Scale (STSSS) was developed by the Shapiros during a clinical trial of Pimozide in the early 1980s, as one of the first instruments measuring changes in tic symptoms. The STSSS is a clinician-rated scale addressing five factors: whether tics are noticeable, if they elicit comments or curiosity, if the patient is considered odd or bizarre, if tics interfere with functioning and if they lead to incapacitation or the patient to be homebound or hospitalized. The item scores can be summed to produce total scores, which are assigned a global severity rating on a 6-point scale from 0 ('no tics') to 6 ('very severe'). The relative simplicity and brevity of the STSSS make it a convenient measure of tic symptoms, taking up to 5 minutes to complete. However, the focus is clearly on tic intensity and interference (plus tic-related social impairment), which somewhat limits the overall accurateness of this clinical assessment of tics. For example, the STSSS does not directly assess tic frequency, complexity or distribution and the time frame within which tic severity is measured is uncertain. The STSSS showed excellent inter-rater reliability (intra-class correlation coefficients by history 0.88, by observation 0.91, overall 0.85; all $p<0.01$) and internal consistency (internal consistency reliability coefficients ranging between 0.82 and 0.97). There was no correlation between the STSSS global severity score and 30-minute videotape tic counts (motor, vocal or total tic counts). When compared with other measures of tic severity, the STSSS showed very good convergent validity with the YGTSS (total tic severity sub-score), the TS-CGI, and the Hopkins Motor and Vocal Tics scale (Spearman's rho correlation coefficients, respectively: by history: 0.85, 0.85, 0.68; by observation: 0.87, 0.76, 0.78; overall: 0.85, 0.87, 0.81). There was also evidence of very good divergent validity with the Obsessive-Compulsive Disorder–Clinical Global Impression and Attention-Deficit Disorder–Clinical Global Impression (Spearman's rho correlation coefficients 0.24 and 0.37, respectively). The STSSS has been successfully used in multiple interventional studies for Tourette syndrome. In 2017, the report of the Committee on Rating Scale Development of the Movement Disorders Society rated the STSSS as a 'recommended' clinician-rated instrument for the assessment of tic severity.

Tourette's Disorder Scale (TODS)

The Tourette's Disorder Scale (TODS) is an objective measure of the severity of tics plus a wide range of Tourette syndrome-related neuropsychiatric symptoms over the period of 1 month. This 15-item instrument contains questions about tics, inattention, hyperactivity, obsessions, compulsions, aggression and emotional symptoms. The items were derived from a questionnaire in which parents were required to rate the occurrence and impact of 32 behavioural and emotional symptoms. Each item is rated between 0 and 10, with five descriptive anchor terms. Clinician- and parent-rated versions are available, both of which have been validated by extensive psychometric testing. The psychometric properties of the clinician-rated and parent-rated versions are similar and the correlation between clinician-rated parent-rated total scores is high. Although the TODS does not assess individual dimensions of tics separately, it has been shown to have adequate psychometric properties. Internal consistency is high for total scores (Cronbach's alpha 0.92 for total parent-rated score and 0.93 for total clinician-rated score), but substantially lower for the tics sub-score (Cronbach's alpha 0.64). Inter-rater reliability is substantial for motor tics (intra-class correlation coefficient 0.79), but variable across the individual scale items for vocal tics (intra-class correlation coefficients ranging between 0.53 and 0.79). Convergent validity with the respective YGTSS sub-scores is moderate for motor tics items (correlation coefficients 0.47 for the clinician-rated version and 0.54 for the parent-rated instrument) and good for vocal tics items (correlation coefficients 0.74 for the clinician-rated version and 0.59 for the parent-rated instrument). The tics sub-score showed low correlation with the obsessive-compulsive and aggression sub-scores. Responsiveness to change of the total score was moderate. Although the administration of the TODS can be time-consuming (about 20 minutes), this scale allows the joint assessment of tics and main co-morbid behavioural features. In 2017, the report of the Committee on Rating Scale Development of the Movement Disorders Society rated the TODS as a 'recommended' clinician-rated instrument for the assessment of tic severity.

Tourette Syndrome–Clinical Global Impression (TS-CGI)

The Clinical Global Impression scale (CGI) is a frequently used measure of disease severity. In preparation for a clinical trial in Tourette syndrome, three disease-specific versions of the CGI were developed (Tourette Syndrome–Clinical Global Impression, TS-CGI). These scales assess symptoms of Tourette syndrome, obsessive-compulsive disorder and attention-deficit and hyperactivity disorder, based on DSM-III diagnostic criteria. The TS-CGI is a clinician-rated seven point ordinal scale that ranks current symptom severity from 'normal' (no identifiable symptoms) to 'extremely severe' (incapacitating tics or high level of functional impairment associated with behavioural symptoms). The TS-CGI shares the same composition with Clinical Global Impression of Severity scales, which are commonly used measures of symptom severity in studies of patients with psychiatric disorders. This instrument rates the overall adverse impact of tics, based on patient and carer interview, and direct examination, rather than assessing individual tic dimensions. The TS-CGI has the advantages of being brief and easy to use: administered in less than 2 minutes, it was used in treatment trials, showing responsiveness to change. The TS-CGI showed excellent inter-rater reliability (intra-class correlation coefficients by history 0.88, by observation 0.83, overall 0.89; all $p<0.01$). When compared with other measures of tic severity, the TS-CGI showed good convergent validity with the YGTSS, the STSSS and the Hopkins Motor and Vocal Tics scale (Spearman's rho correlation coefficients, respectively: by history: 0.84, 0.85, 0.71; by observation: 0.72, 0.76, 0.80; overall: 0.79, 0.87, 0.73). There was also evidence of excellent divergent validity with the Obsessive-Compulsive Disorder–Clinical Global Impression and Attention-Deficit Disorder–Clinical Global Impression (Spearman's rho correlation coefficients 0.23 and 0.40, respectively). In 2017, the report of the Committee on Rating Scale Development of the Movement Disorders Society rated the TS-CGI as a 'recommended' clinician-rated instrument for the assessment of tic severity.

Yale Global Tic Severity Scale (YGTSS)

The Yale Global Tic Severity Scale (YGTSS) is the most widely used clinician-rated measure of tic severity in Tourette syndrome and other tic disorders. The YGTSS is based on a semi-structured interview of symptoms over the past week, where the clinician is asked to record patients' motor and vocal tics. Subsequently, tic severity is rated separately based on tic number, frequency, intensity, complexity and interference on a 6-point Likert-type scale, from 0 ('no tics') to 5 ('severe'), with each point anchored to descriptive statements and relevant examples. The tic severity sub-score consists of the sum of the motor and vocal tic severity scores. In turn, this is summed with the impairment sub-score, which rates the severity of functional impairment from 0 to 50, to produce the YGTSS total score (0–100). The YGTSS allows a multidimensional overview of tic characteristics, as well as the level of functional interference. Factor analytic studies confirmed and validated the scale structure that was initially identified: motor and vocal tics represent two related but separate constructs. The separation of motor and vocal tics is particularly useful for diagnostic purposes. The YGTSS was shown to be characterized by robust psychometric properties, including inter-rater reliability (intra-class correlation coefficients by history 0.94, by observation 0.81, overall 0.93; all $p<0.01$) and internal consistency (Cronbach's alpha: motor tics 0.92, phonic tics 0.93, total tic score 0.93). When compared with other measures of tic severity, the YGTSS showed good convergent validity with the STSSS, the TS-CGI and the Hopkins Motor and Vocal Tics scale (Spearman's rho correlation coefficients, respectively: by history: 0.85, 0.84, 0.71; by observation: 0.87, 0.72, 0.80; overall: 0.85, 0.79, 0.73). There was also evidence of excellent divergent validity with the Obsessive-Compulsive Disorder–Clinical Global Impression and Attention-Deficit Disorder–Clinical Global Impression (Spearman's rho correlation coefficients 0.36 and 0.38, respectively). YGTSS scores showed responsiveness to change in several clinical trials. An important advantage when compared with other instruments is that its total (motor plus vocal) tic severity sub-score has been shown to reliably identify clinically meaningful tic exacerbations. The percentage score reduction considered as best indicator of clinically relevant treatment response varied between 25 per cent and 35 per cent reductions in the tic severity sub-score (and 6–7 points reductions in raw score) across methodologically different studies. The YGTSS is the only rating scale for which cut-off values of score changes indicate clinically relevant exacerbations and treatment responses, making it the most suitable instrument for prospective follow-up in clinic observational longitudinal studies and therapeutic trials. Adaptations of the YGTSS in Korean, Polish, Spanish and Chinese languages have been published. The internal consistency and distribution of the YGTSS scores were examined to inform modification of the measure: the parallel findings across the motor and vocal tic frequency, complexity and interference dimensions prompted minor revisions to the anchor point description to promote use of the full range of scores in each dimension (YGTSS-Revised or YGTSS-R). The YGTSS is an ideal instrument for routine clinical practice, as it takes 15–20 minutes to complete and allows a multidimensional assessment of tic severity and tic-related impairment. In 2017, the report of the Committee on Rating Scale Development of the Movement Disorders Society rated the YGTSS as a 'recommended' clinician-rated instrument for the assessment of tic severity.

Rating Scales for Premonitory Urges

Premonitory Urge for Tics Scales (PUTS and I-PUTS)

The Premonitory Urge of Tics Scale (PUTS) is a relatively brief self-report scale specifically designed to examine premonitory urges in patients with tic disorders. The PUTS was developed based on 10 descriptions of somatic sensations derived from phenomenological accounts reported in the literature and in clinical experience. Although the PUTS originally included 10 items, the item that referred to the ability to actively suppress tics was found to correlate poorly with the total score, and was therefore deleted by the final version of the scale. The severity of urges is rated on a 4-point ordinal scale ('not at all true', 'a little true', 'pretty much true', 'very much true'). Overall psychometric properties were acceptable in older paediatric patients, however initial testing revealed inadequate properties for patients younger than 10 years. Specifically, the PUTS demonstrated high internal consistency for youth older than 10 years (Cronbach's alpha 0.89 in patients aged 11–16 years and 0.83 in patients above 16 years of age, versus 0.57 in patients younger than 10 years). PUTS total scores produced small-to-moderate associations with overall tic severity in some studies, with the findings of other studies suggesting weak or non-significant associations. When examining co-occurring symptoms, a moderate-to-strong relationship was found between PUTS total scores and obsessive-compulsive symptoms, whereas smaller and mixed associations have been reported with overall anxiety symptoms and somatic/panic symptoms. Small associations with affective symptoms have also been identified. There is inconsistent evidence regarding associations between PUTS total scores and measures of ADHD severity, reflecting its variable divergent validity. A correlation between PUTS score and interoceptive awareness has been identified. The results of a study using the PUTS and the University of Sao Paulo Sensory Phenomena Scale showed a statistically significant positive correlation between the total scores of the two instruments (correlation coefficient 0.35). Finally, responsiveness to change of the PUTS is uncertain. A direct translation in Hebrew was presented in a study that provided independent testing of the PUTS showing adequate properties in patients older than 10 years. The PUTS was also translated and validated in Italian. Despite testing in paediatric populations only, adequate psychometric properties for older children and adolescents may indicate utility in adults as well. In 2017, the report of the Committee on Rating Scale Development of the Movement Disorders Society rated the PUTS as a 'recommended' patient-rated instrument for the assessment of sensory phenomena associated with tics in patients older than 10 years.

A newly developed scale, called Individualized PUTS or I-PUTS, provides complementary information to the PUTS. The I-PUTS is a clinician-rated measure that assesses the presence, frequency, intensity and body region location of premonitory urges for individual tics endorsed over the past week, using a symptom checklist that parallels the YGTSS list. For each endorsed tic, the clinician inquires whether a premonitory urge was experienced prior to the tic. Next, the clinician inquires about the frequency of endorsed urges on a 4-point scale from 1 ('urge occurs 0–25% of the time you do the tic') to 4 ('urge occurs 75–100% of the time you do the tic'). The clinician also inquires about the urge intensity on a 4-point scale, from 1 ('minimal intensity/urge can be ignored for a considerable amount of time') to 4 ('strong intensity/urge needs relief almost immediately'). Finally, the clinician enquires about the body region associated with each urge, based on six anatomical categories: head/face, neck/throat, torso, arms, legs and whole body/other. The items are summed to create a total number of distinct urges (I-PUTS Urge Number), total urge frequency (I-PUTS Frequency) and total urge intensity (I-PUTS Intensity). According to the results of the I-PUTS development and validation study, young patients with Tourette syndrome and other tic disorders experienced an average of three distinct urges, but had an average of seven tics over a week prior to data collection. Premonitory urges were primarily localized in the head/face, neck/throat and arm regions. All I-PUTS dimensions were characterized by excellent inter-rater reliability (inter-class correlation coefficients 0.83 for Urge Number, 0.76 for Urge Frequency and 0.87 for Urge Intensity). The I-PUTS dimensions also exhibited good convergent validity with global urge ratings (PUTS) and tic severity (YGTSS), and appropriate divergent validity from other clinical constructs (no significant associations with measures of depression, rage, obsessive-compulsive symptoms, attention problems, dysregulation and/or other internalizing or externalizing behaviours).

Rating Scales for Quality of Life

Gilles de la Tourette Syndrome–Quality of Life Scales (GTS-QOL, C&A-GTS-QOL)

The concept of health-related quality of life is of paramount importance in determining the impact of Tourette syndrome and other tic disorders on patients' experiences of everyday life. Specifically, an accurate measurement of perceived quality of life is particularly useful as it covers all aspects of disease burden and allows subjective perspectives to be captured. There is a need for reliable and valid psychometric instruments assessing quality of life in a holistic sense across both cross-sectional or longitudinal studies, particularly when investigating potential therapeutic strategies. Over the last few decades, a number of disease-specific quality of life scales have become available for a wide range of neuropsychiatric conditions. The Gilles de la Tourette Syndrome–Quality of Life Scale (GTS-QOL) was the first quality of life measure specifically developed for patients with Tourette syndrome. The items included in this scale were derived from exploratory studies aimed at capturing clinically relevant issues through semi-structured patient interviews, consultation with experts and literature reviews. After the item generation stage, an item pool of 102 questions was reduced to 40 questions by deleting duplicates and inappropriate items and grouping related questions. Further reductions to the questionnaire were suggested by the results of a principal component analysis to produce the final 27-item instrument. The GTS-QOL has a four-factor structure covering four domains: the 'psychological' domain, with 11 items addressing the burden of affective and anxiety symptoms; the 'physical and activities of daily living' domain, with 7 items addressing functional impairment due to motor dyscontrol; the 'obsessive-compulsive' domain, with 5 items addressing the impact of obsessive-compulsive symptoms; the 'cognitive' domain, with 4 items addressing the consequences of memory and concentration problems. Each item is rated on a 5-point Likert-like scale from 0 ('no problem') to 4 ('extreme problem'), and a 0–100 visual analogue scale is included to estimate overall satisfaction with life. Psychometric evaluations demonstrated that the GTS-QOL is a valid and reliable disease-specific instrument for the assessment of quality of life in adult patient with Tourette syndrome. Specifically, the GTS-QOL was shown to be characterized by high internal consistency reliability and test-retest reliability (Cronbach's alpha values above 0.8 and intra-class correlation coefficients above 0.8); validity was supported by inter-scale correlations (range 0.5–0.7), confirmatory factor analysis, and correlation patterns with other rating scales (including the MOVES) and clinical variables. The GTS-QOL has been used in multiple clinical studies, including treatment interventions of different kinds, as an adjunct measure to tic severity ratings to capture the patients' perception of their overall quality of life. This psychometric instrument has also allowed the assessment of predictors during childhood of future quality of life in adult patients and the relative impact of premonitory urges and behavioural co-morbidities on quality of life in Tourette syndrome.

A multicentre study conducted in Italy led to the translation, adaptation and validation of the GTS-QOL for young Italian patients with Tourette syndrome. The Gilles de la Tourette Syndrome–Quality of Life Scale in children and adolescents (C&A-GTS-QOL) is a 27-item instrument for the assessment of quality of life through a clinician-rated interview for 6- to 12-year-olds and a self-report questionnaire for 13- to 18-year-olds. The first disease-specific quality of life rating scale for young patients with Tourette syndrome demonstrated satisfactory internal consistency reliability (Cronbach's alpha values for all sub-scales exceeded 0.7), internal construct validity (moderate correlation between the sub-scale scores), and convergent and divergent validity (correlations with other scales and variables known to influence quality of life). The Italian version of the C&A-GTS-QOL was used in multiple studies on clinical samples from Italy. Following language adaptation from Italian to English language, standard statistical methods were used to test the psychometric properties of the English version of the C&A-GTS-QOL in the UK. Principal component factor analyses led to the identification of six quality of life domains (cognitive, coprophenomena, psychological, physical, obsessive-compulsive and activities of daily living), explaining 66.7 per cent of the overall variance. The English version of the C&A-GTS-QOL demonstrated satisfactory internal consistency reliability (Cronbach's alpha values ranging from 0.5 to 0.9 across the six sub-scales), whereas validity was supported by inter-scale correlations, confirmatory factor analysis and correlation patterns with other rating scales (including the MOVES) and relevant clinical variables.

Chapter

3

First-Generation Anti-dopaminergic Medications

Fluphenazine

Pharmacological Properties

The main pharmacodynamic and pharmacokinetic properties of Fluphenazine (Figure 3.1) are summarized in Table 3.1.

Figure 3.1 Fluphenazine.

Table 3.1 Main pharmacodynamic and pharmacokinetic properties of Fluphenazine

Mechanism(s) of action

Antagonism of D1 and D2 dopamine receptors

Antagonism of 5-HT1A, 5-HT2A, 5-HT2C, 5-HT7 serotonin receptors

Antagonism of alpha-1A and alpha-2 adrenergic receptors

Antagonism of H1 histaminergic receptors

Antagonism of M1 muscarinic cholinergic receptors

Pharmacokinetics

Peak effect at variable times

Elimination half-life of approximately 15 hours

Eliminated in both urine and faeces

Preparations

The relevant medicinal forms of Fluphenazine are shown in Table 3.2.

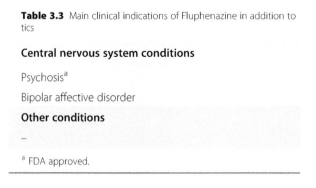

Table 3.2 Relevant medicinal forms of Fluphenazine

Tablets

Fluphenazine 1 mg

Fluphenazine 2.5 mg

Fluphenazine 5 mg

Fluphenazine 10 mg

Oral solution[a]

Fluphenazine 2.5 mg/5 ml

Fluphenazine 5 mg/1 ml (concentrate)

[a] Oral solution should not be mixed with drinks containing caffeine, tannic acid (tea), pectinates (apple juice).

Dose Titration

Dose is 1–2.5 mg daily for 14 days, then increased by 1–2.5 mg every 14 days; usual maintenance 10–20 mg daily in two divided doses (maximum dose 40 mg daily).

Other Indications

The main clinical indications of Fluphenazine in addition to tics are listed in Table 3.3.

Table 3.3 Main clinical indications of Fluphenazine in addition to tics

Central nervous system conditions

Psychosis[a]

Bipolar affective disorder

Other conditions

—

[a] FDA approved.

Cautions

Caution is warranted when using Fluphenazine in patients with the conditions listed in Table 3.4.

Table 3.4 Cautions about the use of Fluphenazine

Central nervous system conditions

Central nervous system depression[a]

Parkinson disease[a], Lewy body dementia[a]

Seizures

Other conditions

Co-administration of Cabergoline, Metrizamide, Pergolide[a]

[a] Contraindication.

Adverse Effects

The overall tolerability of Fluphenazine in terms of sedation and weight gain is shown in Table 3.5, whereas the frequency of individual adverse effects is presented in Table 3.6.

Table 3.5 Overall tolerability of Fluphenazine in terms of sedation and weight gain

Sedation	☹
Weight gain	☹

☹☹☹ = significant problem
☹☹ = frequently reported
☹ = occasionally reported

Table 3.6 Frequency of adverse effects associated with Fluphenazine

Very common (>1 in 10 patients on Fluphenazine)	
CENTRAL NERVOUS SYSTEM:	OTHER SYSTEMS:
– Akathisia	–
– Extrapyramidal symptoms	
– Rigidity	
– Tardive dyskinesias/dystonia	
– Tremor	
Common (>1 in 100 patients on Fluphenazine)	
CENTRAL NERVOUS SYSTEM:	OTHER SYSTEMS:
– Depression	– Blurred vision
– Dizziness	– Constipation
– Sedation	– Dry eyes
	– Dry mouth

Table 3.6 (cont.)

Common (>1 in 100 patients on Fluphenazine)

- Hypotension
- Syncope
- Tachycardia
- Urinary retention
- Weight gain

Uncommon (>1 in 1000 patients on Fluphenazine)

CENTRAL NERVOUS SYSTEM:	OTHER SYSTEMS:
– Neuroleptic malignant syndrome	– Agranulocytosis
	– Amenorrhoea
	– Electrocardiogram abnormalities
	– Thromboembolism
	– Galactorrhoea
	– Gynaecomastia
	– Hyperprolactinaemia
	– Sexual dysfunction

Rare (>1 in 10,000 patients on Fluphenazine)

CENTRAL NERVOUS SYSTEM:	OTHER SYSTEMS:
– Seizures	– Hypercholesterolaemia
	– Jaundice
	– Priapism
	– Skin disorders

Very rare (<1 in 10 000 patients on Fluphenazine)

CENTRAL NERVOUS SYSTEM:	OTHER SYSTEMS:
–	– Anti-nuclear antibodies
	– Systemic lupus erythematosus

Interactions

The most relevant clinical interactions between Fluphenazine and alcohol/other medications are shown in Table 3.7.

Table 3.7 Most relevant clinical interactions between Fluphenazine and alcohol/other medications

Agent	Effect
Adrenaline	Concomitant administration of Fluphenazine and Adrenaline may increase the risk of hypotension.
Alcohol	Concomitant administration of Fluphenazine and alcohol may increase the risk of hypotension.
Anti-hypertensive medications	Fluphenazine may increase their effects (except Guanethidine, whose effects Fluphenazine may antagonize).

Table 3.7 (cont.)

Agent	Effect
Atropine and related medications	Concomitant administration of Fluphenazine and Atropine (or related medications) may result in additive anti-cholinergic effects.
Diuretics	Concomitant administration of Fluphenazine and diuretics may increase the risk of hypotension.
Levodopa and dopamine-agonists	Fluphenazine may decrease their effects.
Lithium	Concomitant administration of Fluphenazine and Lithium may increase the risk of encephalopathic syndrome similar to neuroleptic malignant syndrome.

Special Populations

The main recommendations for the use of Fluphenazine in patients with hepatic and renal impairment are shown in Table 3.8.

Table 3.8 Main recommendations for the use of Fluphenazine in patients with hepatic and renal impairment

Hepatic impairment	Use with caution (slower titration is recommended).
Renal impairment	Use with caution (slower titration is recommended).

The main recommendations for the use of Fluphenazine during pregnancy and breast-feeding are shown in Table 3.9.

Table 3.9 Main recommendations for the use of Fluphenazine during pregnancy and breastfeeding

Pregnancy	Animal reproduction studies have shown adverse effects on the foetus, and there are no controlled studies in humans, but potential benefits may warrant use of the medication in pregnant women despite potential risks of extrapyramidal symptoms, jaundice, hyper/hyporeflexia. Overall, there is a risk of abnormal movements and withdrawal symptoms (agitation, hyper/hypotonia, tremor, sedation, breathing and/or feeding problems) in newborns whose mothers took an anti-dopaminergic medication during the third semester (former FDA Pregnancy Category C).
Breastfeeding	A small amount is present in breast milk: avoid due to risk of sedation, dystonia and tardive dyskinesias.

Behavioural Neurology

Fluphenazine is a high-potency phenotiazine characterized by lower risk of sedation and hypotension but higher risk of extrapyramidal adverse effects compared to low-potency phenotiazines. There is considerable evidence about the efficacy of Fluphenazine in both psychotic and affective disorders. This medication is sometimes administered to patients with motor and autonomic hyperactivity, as well as agitation and aggressive behaviours, with tolerability being the main limiting factor for a more widespread use. Moreover,

Fluphenazine was not shown to be effective for behavioural problems in patients with learning difficulties. The evidence supporting its effectiveness on tics (and other hyperkinetic conditions) is overall weaker compared to other first-generation anti-dopaminergic medications.

Guidelines

The main recommendations for the use of Fluphenazine according to the clinical guidelines on the treatment of tics are shown in Table 3.10.

Table 3.10 Main recommendations for the use of Fluphenazine according to published guidelines on the treatment of tics

Country (year)	Recommendation about Fluphenazine	Population
EU (+UK) (2011)	Listed as an additional first-generation anti-dopaminergic agent used particularly in the US; not included in top three recommendations in survey of preferred choices	Children + adults
EU (+UK) (2012)[a]	Not included in top three recommendations	Children + adults
Canada (2012)	Weak recommendation, low-quality evidence	Children + adults
US (2013)	Listed with comments on risk of extrapyramidal symptoms lower than with Haloperidol	Children
UK (2016)	Not listed	Children
Japan (2019)[a]	Not included as first/second choice	Children + adults
US (2019)	Listed as an additional first-generation anti-dopaminergic agent for which evidence is promising but limited	Children + adults

[a] Expert survey and consensus.

Overall Rating

A summary of the efficacy and tolerability profiles of Fluphenazine in patients with Tourette syndrome is presented in Table 3.11.

Table 3.11 Summary of efficacy and tolerability profiles of Fluphenazine in patients with Tourette syndrome

Efficacy for tics	☺
Efficacy for behavioural problems	☺
Tolerability	☺

☺☺☺ = very good
☺☺ = good
☺ = acceptable

Haloperidol

Pharmacological Properties

The main pharmacodynamic and pharmacokinetic properties of Haloperidol (Figure 3.2) are summarized in Table 3.12.

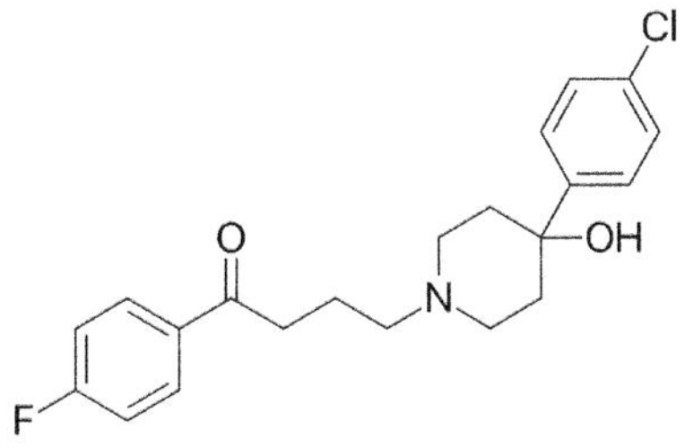

Figure 3.2 Haloperidol.

Table 3.12 Main pharmacodynamic and pharmacokinetic properties of Haloperidol

Mechanism(s) of action

Antagonism of D2, D3, D4 dopamine receptors

Antagonism of 5-HT1A, 5-HT2A, 5-HT2C, 5-HT7 serotonin receptors

Antagonism of alpha-1A and alpha-2 adrenergic receptors

Antagonism of H1 histaminergic receptors

Antagonism of M1 muscarinic cholinergic receptors

Pharmacokinetics

Peak effect in approximately 4 hours

Elimination half-life of approximately 24 hours

Eliminated in both urine and faeces

Preparations

The relevant medicinal forms of Haloperidol are shown in Table 3.13.

Table 3.13 Relevant medicinal forms of Haloperidol

Tablets

Haloperidol 0.5 mg

Haloperidol 1.5 mg

Haloperidol 5 mg

Haloperidol 10 mg

Table 3.13 (cont.)

Capsules

Haloperidol 0.5 mg

Oral solution

Haloperidol 5 mg/5 ml

Haloperidol 10 mg/5 ml

Dose Titration

Dose is 0.5–1 mg daily for 14 days, then increased by 0.5–1 mg every 14 days; usual maintenance 1.5–3 mg daily in one to three divided doses (maximum dose 6–9 mg daily; safety not established for doses over 100 mg daily).

Other Indications

The main clinical indications of Haloperidol in addition to tics are listed in Table 3.14.

Table 3.14 Main clinical indications of Haloperidol in addition to tics

Central nervous system conditions

Irritability and aggressiveness[a]

Psychosis[a]

Bipolar affective disorder

Delirium

Obsessive-compulsive disorder (augmentation therapy)

Other conditions

Nausea

[a] FDA approved.

Cautions

Caution is warranted when using Haloperidol in patients with the conditions listed in Table 3.15.

Adverse Effects

The overall tolerability of Haloperidol in terms of sedation and weight gain is shown in Table 3.16, whereas the frequency of individual adverse effects is presented in Table 3.17.

Table 3.15 Cautions about the use of Haloperidol

Central nervous system conditions

Central nervous system depression[a]

Parkinson disease[a], Lewy body dementia[a], Progressive supranuclear palsy[a]

Risk factors for stroke

Other conditions

Congenital long QT syndrome and QT interval prolongation[a], history of torsade de pointes[a], history of ventricular arrhythmias[a], recent acute myocardial infarction[a], uncompensated heart failure[a]

Hypokalaemia[a]

Bradycardia, family history of QT interval prolongation

Electrolyte disturbances

History of heavy alcohol exposure

Hyperprolactinaemia and prolactin-dependent tumours

Hyperthyroidism

Hypotension

[a] Contraindication.

Table 3.16 Overall tolerability of Haloperidol in terms of sedation and weight gain

Sedation	☹☹
Weight gain	☹

☹☹☹ = significant problem
☹☹ = frequently reported
☹ = occasionally reported

Table 3.17 Frequency of adverse effects associated with Haloperidol

Very common (>1 in 10 patients on Haloperidol)	
CENTRAL NERVOUS SYSTEM:	OTHER SYSTEMS:
– Agitation	–
– Extrapyramidal symptoms	
– Headache	
– Hyperkinesias	
– Insomnia	
Common (>1 in 100 patients on Haloperidol)	
CENTRAL NERVOUS SYSTEM:	OTHER SYSTEMS:
– Akathisia	– Constipation
– Bradykinesia	– Dry mouth
– Depression	– Erectile dysfunction

Table 3.17 (cont.)

Common (>1 in 100 patients on Haloperidol)

- Dizziness
- Dyskinesias
- Dystonia
- Hypertonia
- Hypokinesia
- Oculogyric crisis
- Psychosis
- Somnolence
- Tardive dyskinesias
- Tremor
- Hypersalivation
- Hypotension
- Liver enzyme abnormalities
- Nausea and vomiting
- Skin rash
- Urinary retention
- Visual disturbances
- Weight changes

Uncommon (>1 in 1000 patients on Haloperidol)

CENTRAL NERVOUS SYSTEM:

- Akinesia
- Confusion
- Decreased libido
- Gait problems
- Restlessness
- Sedation
- Seizures

OTHER SYSTEMS:

- Amenorrhoea and dysmenorrhoea
- Blurred vision
- Breast discomfort/pain
- Dyspnoea
- Galactorrhoea
- Hepatitis
- Hyperhydrosis
- Hyperthermia
- Jaundice
- Leukopenia
- Muscle spasms and rigidity
- Oedema
- Photosensitivity reaction
- Pruritus
- Tachycardia
- Torticollis

Rare (>1 in 10 000 patients on Haloperidol)

CENTRAL NERVOUS SYSTEM:

- Neuroleptic malignant syndrome
- Nystagmus

OTHER SYSTEMS:

- Bronchospasm
- Hyperprolactinaemia
- Menstrual disorder
- QT prolongation
- Sexual dysfunction
- Trismus

Very rare (<1 in 10 000 patients on Haloperidol)

CENTRAL NERVOUS SYSTEM:

-

OTHER SYSTEMS:

-

Interactions

The most relevant clinical interactions between Haloperidol and alcohol/other medications are shown in Table 3.18.

Table 3.18 Most relevant clinical interactions between Haloperidol and alcohol/other medications

Agent	Effect
Adrenaline	Concomitant administration of Haloperidol and Adrenaline may increase the risk of hypotension.
Alcohol	Concomitant administration of Haloperidol and alcohol may increase the risk of central nervous system depression.
Anticoagulants	Haloperidol may decrease their effects.
Anti-hypertensive medications	Haloperidol may increase their effects (except Guanethidine, whose effects Haloperidol may antagonize).
Atropine and related medications	Concomitant administration of Haloperidol and Atropine (or related medications) may result in additive anti-cholinergic effects.
Levodopa and dopamine-agonists	Haloperidol may decrease their effects.
Lithium	Concomitant administration of Haloperidol and Lithium may increase the risk of encephalopathic syndrome similar to neuroleptic malignant syndrome.
Rifampin	Plasma levels of Haloperidol may be lowered.

Special Populations

The main recommendations for the use of Haloperidol in patients with hepatic and renal impairment are shown in Table 3.19.

Table 3.19 Main recommendations for the use of Haloperidol in patients with hepatic and renal impairment

Hepatic impairment	Use with caution (halve initial dose and adjust if necessary with smaller increments and at longer intervals).
Renal impairment	Use with caution (consider lower initial dose in severe impairment and adjust if necessary with smaller increments and at longer intervals).

The main recommendations for the use of Haloperidol during pregnancy and breast-feeding are shown in Table 3.20.

Table 3.20 Main recommendations for the use of Haloperidol during pregnancy and breastfeeding

Pregnancy	Animal reproduction studies have shown adverse effects on the foetus, and there are no controlled studies in humans, but potential benefits may warrant use of the medication in pregnant women despite potential risks of extrapyramidal symptoms, jaundice, hyper/hyporeflexia and limb deformity. Overall, there is a risk of abnormal movements and withdrawal symptoms (agitation, hyper/hypotonia, tremor, sedation, breathing and/or feeding problems) in newborns whose mothers took an anti-dopaminergic medication during the third semester (former FDA Pregnancy Category C).
Breastfeeding	A small amount is present in breast milk: use while breastfeeding is not recommended.

Behavioural Neurology

Haloperidol is mainly used as an anti-psychotic medication, although it is not clearly effective for the cognitive or affective symptoms of schizophrenia. It is sometimes also used for the maintenance treatment of bipolar affective disorder, despite the risk of developing tardive dyskinesias. Overall, Haloperidol is less sedating than other first-generation anti-dopaminergic medications. Haloperidol was the first medication found to be effective in the treatment of tics and still is one of the most powerful anti-tic agents. Haloperidol was also the first medication approved by the FDA for the treatment of adults (1969) and children (1978) with Tourette syndrome. More recently, the availability of better tolerated tic-suppressing agents has led to a considerable decrease in its use, which is currently limited by its adverse effect profile.

Guidelines

The main recommendations for the use of Haloperidol according to the clinical guidelines on the treatment of tics are shown in Table 3.21.

Table 3.21 Main recommendations for the use of Haloperidol according to published guidelines on the treatment of tics

Country (year)	Recommendation about Haloperidol	Population
EU (+UK) (2011)	Evidence Level A; included as seventh medication in survey of preferred choices	Children + adults
EU (+UK) (2012)[a]	Not included in top three recommendations	Children + adults
Canada (2012)	Weak recommendation, high-quality evidence	Children + adults
US (2013)	Listed with comments on adverse effects (extrapyramidal symptoms, reports of anxiety flares) (FDA-approved indication for Tourette syndrome)	Children
UK (2016)	Low certainty in the effect estimate (children + adults) (downgraded because of suboptimal sample size and high risk of bias)	Children

Table 3.21 (cont.)

Country (year)	Recommendation about Haloperidol	Population
Japan (2019)*	Included as second choice	Children + adults
US (2019)	Moderate certainty in the effect estimate (children + adults) (based on two Class II studies)	Children + adults

[a] Expert survey and consensus

Overall Rating

A summary of the efficacy and tolerability profiles of Haloperidol in patients with Tourette syndrome is presented in Table 3.22.

Table 3.22 Summary of efficacy and tolerability profiles of Haloperidol in patients with Tourette syndrome

Efficacy for tics	☺☺☺
Efficacy for behavioural problems	☺
Tolerability	☺

☺☺☺ = very good
☺☺ = good
☺ = acceptable

Pimozide

Pharmacological Properties

The main pharmacodynamic and pharmacokinetic properties of Pimozide (Figure 3.3) are summarized in Table 3.23.

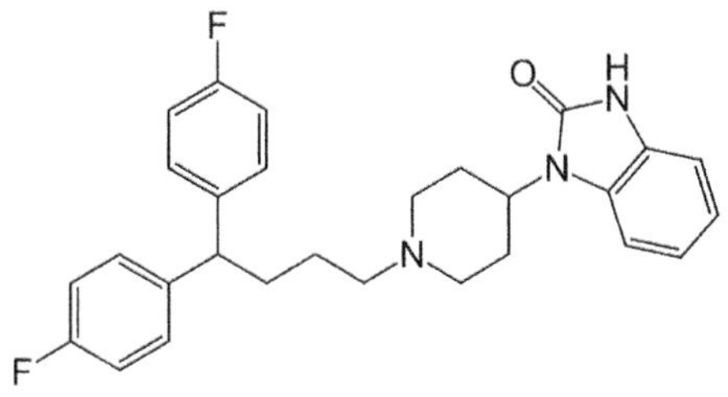

Figure 3.3 Pimozide.

Preparations

The relevant medicinal forms of Pimozide are shown in Table 3.24.

Table 3.23 Main pharmacodynamic and pharmacokinetic properties of Pimozide

Mechanism(s) of action

Antagonism of D2, D3, D4 dopamine receptors

Antagonism of 5-HT1A, 5-HT2A, 5-HT2C, 5-HT7 serotonin receptors

Antagonism of alpha-1A and alpha-2 adrenergic receptors

Antagonism of H1 histaminergic receptors

Antagonism of M1 muscarinic cholinergic receptors

Blockade of calcium channels

Blockade of hERG (human ether-a-go-go-related gene)

Pharmacokinetics

Peak effect at variable times

Elimination half-life of approximately 55 hours

Eliminated mainly in urine (after extensive liver metabolism, mainly by CYP450 3A)

Table 3.24 Relevant medicinal forms of Pimozide

Tablets

Pimozide 1 mg

Pimozide 2 mg

Pimozide 4 mg

Dose Titration

Dose is 1 mg daily for 14 days, then increased by 1 mg every 14 days; usual maintenance 2–10 mg daily in one to two divided doses (maximum dose 20 mg daily).

Other Indications

The main clinical indications of Pimozide in addition to tics are listed in Table 3.25.

Table 3.25 Main clinical indications of Pimozide in addition to tics

Central nervous system conditions

Psychosis

Other conditions

–

*FDA-approved

Cautions

Caution is warranted when using Pimozide in patients with the conditions listed in Table 3.26.

Table 3.26 Cautions about the use of Pimozide

Central nervous system conditions

Central nervous system depression[a]

Parkinson disease, Lewy body dementia

Other conditions

History of arrhythmias[a], recent acute myocardial infarction[a], uncompensated heart failure[a], history or family history of congenital QT prolongation[a], co-administration of medications capable of prolonging the QT interval (e.g. selected anti-arrhythmics, Moxifloxacine, Sparfloxacin, Thioridazine, Ziprasidone)[a]

Phaeochromocytoma[a]

Bradycardia (incl. induced by beta blockers, calcium channel blockers, Clonidine, digitalis)

Co-administration of medications that cause electrolyte disturbances (e.g. diuretics)

Co-administration of medications that inhibit Pimozide metabolism (e.g. azole anti-fungal agents, Fluoxetine, Fluvoxamine, macrolide antibiotics, Nefazodone, protease inhibitors, Sertraline)

Hypokalaemia and/or hypomagnesaemia (incl. induced by diuretics, stimulant laxatives, intravenous Amphoterin B, glucocorticoids, Tetracosactide)

[a] Contraindication.

Adverse Effects

The overall tolerability of Pimozide in terms of sedation and weight gain is shown in Table 3.27, whereas the frequency of individual adverse effects is presented in Table 3.28.

Table 3.27 Overall tolerability of Pimozide in terms of sedation and weight gain

Sedation	☹☹
Weight gain	☹☹

☹☹☹ = significant problem
☹☹ = frequently reported
☹ = occasionally reported

Interactions

The most relevant clinical interactions between Pimozide and alcohol/other medications are shown in Table 3.29.

Table 3.28 Frequency of adverse effects associated with Pimozide

Very common (>1 in 10 patients on Pimozide)

CENTRAL NERVOUS SYSTEM:

– Dizziness
– Sedation

OTHER SYSTEMS:

– Hyperhidrosis
– Nocturia

Common (>1 in 100 patients on Pimozide)

CENTRAL NERVOUS SYSTEM:

– Agitation
– Akathisia
– Depression
– Extrapyramidal symptoms
– Fatigue
– Headache
– Insomnia
– Muscle rigidity
– Restlessness
– Tremor

OTHER SYSTEMS:

– Anorexia
– Blurred vision
– Constipation
– Dry mouth
– Erectile dysfunction
– Hypersalivation
– Nausea and vomiting
– Sebaceous gland overactivity
– Urinary frequency
– Weight gain

Uncommon (>1 in 1000 patients on Pimozide)

CENTRAL NERVOUS SYSTEM:

– Bradykinesia
– Dyskinesias
– Dystonia
– Dysarthria
– Rigidity

OTHER SYSTEMS:

– Amenorrhoea
– Face oedema
– Muscle spasms
– Skin reactions

Rare (>1 in 10 000 patients on Pimozide)

CENTRAL NERVOUS SYSTEM:

– Neuroleptic malignant syndrome
– Seizures

OTHER SYSTEMS:

– Galactorrhoea
– Gynaecomastia
– Hyperglycaemia
– Hyponatraemia

Very rare (<1 in 10 000 patients on Pimozide)

CENTRAL NERVOUS SYSTEM:

–

OTHER SYSTEMS:

– QT prolongation, torsade de pointes, ventricular arrhythmias

Special Populations

The main recommendations for the use of Pimozide in patients with hepatic and renal impairment are shown in Table 3.30.

The main recommendations for the use of Pimozide during pregnancy and breastfeeding are shown in Table 3.31.

Table 3.29 Most relevant clinical interactions between Pimozide and alcohol/other medications

Agent	Effect
Adrenaline	Concomitant administration of Pimozide and Adrenaline may increase the risk of hypotension.
Alcohol	Concomitant administration of Pimozide and alcohol may increase the risk of central nervous system depression.
Anti-hypertensive medications	Pimozide may increase their effects.
CYP450 3A4 inhibitors (e.g. Fluoxetine, Fluvoxamine, Nefazodone, Sertraline, grapefruit juice)	Concomitant administration of Pimozide and CYP450 3A4 inhibitors may result in raised Pimozide levels and increased risk of arrhythmias.
Fluoxetine	Concomitant administration of Pimozide and Fluoxetine may increase the risk for bradycardia.
Levodopa and dopamine-agonists	Pimozide may decrease their effects.
Lithium	Concomitant administration of Pimozide and Lithium may increase the risk of encephalopathic syndrome similar to neuroleptic malignant syndrome.
Medications capable of prolonging the QT interval (e.g. selected anti-arrhythmics, Moxifloxacin, Sparfloxacin, Thioridazine, Ziprasidone)	Concomitant administration of Pimozide and medications capable of significantly prolonging the QT interval may increase the risk of arrhythmias.

Table 3.30 Main recommendations for the use of Pimozide in patients with hepatic and renal impairment

Hepatic impairment	Use with caution, as it can precipitate coma.
Renal impairment	Use with caution (start with small doses in patients with severe renal impairment because of increased cerebral sensitivity).

Table 3.31 Main recommendations for the use of Pimozide during pregnancy and breastfeeding

Pregnancy	Animal reproduction studies have shown adverse effects on the foetus and there are no controlled studies in humans, but potential benefits may warrant use of the medication in pregnant women despite potential risks of extrapyramidal symptoms, jaundice, hyper/hyporeflexia and renal papillary abnormalities. Overall, there is a risk of abnormal movements and withdrawal symptoms (agitation, hyper/hypotonia, tremor, sedation, breathing and/or feeding problems) in newborns whose mothers took an anti-dopaminergic medication during the third semester (former FDA Pregnancy Category C).
Breastfeeding	It is unknown if Pimozide is secreted in breast milk: its use while breastfeeding is not recommended because of potential for tumorigenicity or cardiovascular effects on newborn.

Behavioural Neurology

In addition to psychosis (positive symptoms), Pimozide has previously been used for the treatment of selected behavioural problems, including monosymptomatic hypochondriasis. It is no longer recommended for use in any other neurodevelopmental condition than Tourette syndrome. Although in the past Pimozide was considered a first-line choice for the treatment of tics, it is currently recognized that its benefits generally do not outweigh its associated risks in most patients. Therefore it is currently used as pharmacotherapy of tics in patients who failed to respond to other treatment interventions. In consideration of its potential cardiotoxicity (dose-dependent effects on the QT interval), baseline and repeated electrocardiograms and potassium levels (e.g. at dose changes) are recommended.

Guidelines

The main recommendations for the use of Pimozide according to the clinical guidelines on the treatment of tics are shown in Table 3.32.

Table 3.32 Main recommendations for the use of Pimozide according to published guidelines on the treatment of tics

Country (year)	Recommendation about Pimozide	Population
EU (+UK) (2011)	Evidence Level A; included as fourth medication in survey of preferred choices	Children + adults
EU (+UK) (2012)[a]	Not included in top three recommendations	Children + adults
Canada (2012)	Weak recommendation, high-quality evidence	Children + adults
US (2013)	Listed with comments on adverse effects (recommended ECG monitoring) (FDA-approved indication for Tourette syndrome)	Children
UK (2016)	Low certainty in the effect estimate (children) (downgraded because of suboptimal sample size and high risk of bias)	Children
Japan (2019)[a]	Not included as first/second choice	Children + adults
US (2019)	Low certainty in the effect estimate (children + adults) (based on three Class II studies – confidence in evidence downgraded due to imprecision)	Children + adults

[a] Expert survey and consensus.

Overall Rating

A summary of the efficacy and tolerability profiles of Pimozide in patients with Tourette syndrome is presented in Table 3.33.

Table 3.33 Summary of efficacy and tolerability profiles of Pimozide in patients with Tourette syndrome

Efficacy for tics	☺☺☺
Efficacy for behavioural problems	☺
Tolerability	☺

☺☺☺ = very good
☺☺ = good
☺ = acceptable

Second-Generation Anti-dopaminergic Medications

Aripiprazole

Pharmacological Properties

The main pharmacodynamic and pharmacokinetic properties of Aripiprazole (Figure 4.1) are summarized in Table 4.1.

Figure 4.1 Aripiprazole.

Table 4.1 Main pharmacodynamic and pharmacokinetic properties of Aripiprazole

Mechanism(s) of action

Partial agonism of D2 and D3 dopamine receptors

Partial agonism of 5-HT1A serotonin receptors

Antagonism of 5-HT1D, 5-HT2A, 5-HT2B, 5-HT2C, 5-HT7 serotonin receptors

Antagonism of alpha-1, alpha-2A and alpha-2C adrenergic receptors

Antagonism of H1 histaminergic receptors

Pharmacokinetics

Peak effect in approximately 3–5 hours

Elimination half-life of approximately 75 hours

Eliminated mainly in the faeces (after extensive liver metabolism, mainly by CYP450 2D6 and CYP450 3A4)

Preparations

The relevant medicinal forms of Aripiprazole are shown in Table 4.2.

Table 4.2 Relevant medicinal forms of Aripiprazole

Tablets

Aripiprazole 5 mg

Aripiprazole 10 mg

Aripiprazole 15 mg

Aripiprazole 30 mg

Oral solution

Aripiprazole 1 mg/1 ml

Dose Titration

Dose is 2.5–5 mg daily for 14 days, then increased by 5 mg every 14 days; usual maintenance 10–20 mg once daily (maximum dose 30 mg daily).

Other Indications

The main clinical indications of Aripiprazole in addition to tics are listed in Table 4.3.

Table 4.3 Main clinical indications of Aripiprazole in addition to tics

Central nervous system conditions

Psychosis[a]

Bipolar affective disorder[a]

Depression (adjunctive therapy)[a]

Irritability and aggressiveness

Obsessive-compulsive disorder (augmentation therapy)

Anxiety

Other conditions

–

[a] FDA approved.

Cautions

Caution is warranted when using Aripiprazole in patients with the conditions listed in Table 4.4.

Adverse Effects

The overall tolerability of Aripiprazole in terms of sedation and weight gain is shown in Table 4.5, whereas the frequency of individual adverse effects is presented in Table 4.6.

Table 4.4 Cautions about the use of Aripiprazole

Central nervous system conditions

Central nervous system depression[a]

Other conditions

Phaeochromocytoma[a]

Cerebrovascular disease

[a] Contraindication.

Table 4.5 Overall tolerability of Aripiprazole in terms of sedation and weight gain

Sedation	☺
Weight gain	☺

☹☹☹ = significant problem
☹☹ = frequently reported
☹ = occasionally reported

Table 4.6 Frequency of adverse effects associated with Aripiprazole

Very common (>1 in 10 patients on Aripiprazole)	
CENTRAL NERVOUS SYSTEM:	OTHER SYSTEMS:
–	–

Common (>1 in 100 patients on Aripiprazole)	
CENTRAL NERVOUS SYSTEM:	OTHER SYSTEMS:
– Akathisia	– Blurred vision
– Anxiety	– Constipation
– Dizziness	– Diabetes mellitus
– Extrapyramidal symptoms	– Dyspepsia
– Fatigue	– Hypersalivation
– Headache	– Nausea and vomiting
– Insomnia	
– Restlessness	
– Sedation	
– Tremor	

Uncommon (>1 in 1000 patients on Aripiprazole)	
CENTRAL NERVOUS SYSTEM:	OTHER SYSTEMS:
– Depression	– Diplopia
– Dystonia	– Hiccups
– Hypersexuality	– Hyperglycaemia
– Tardive dyskinesias	– Hyperprolactinaemia
	– Hypotension
	– Tachycardia

Table 4.6 (cont.)

Rare (>1 in 10 000 patients on Aripiprazole)	
CENTRAL NERVOUS SYSTEM:	OTHER SYSTEMS:
– Impulse control disorders	– Alopecia
	– Bradycardia, QT prolongation, torsade de pointes, ventricular arrhythmias
	– Diarrhoea
	– Dysphagia
	– Chest pain
	– Hyperhidorsis
	– Hyperglycaemia
	– Hypertension
	– Jaundice
	– Laryngospasm/oropharyngeal spasm
	– Liver enzyme abnormalities
	– Myalgia
	– Oedema
	– Priapism
	– Skin reactions
	– Stiffness
	– Syncope
	– Temperature dysregulation
	– Thromboembolism
	– Urinary incontinence/ retention
Very rare (<1 in 10 000 patients on Aripiprazole)	
CENTRAL NERVOUS SYSTEM:	OTHER SYSTEMS:
–	–

Interactions

The most relevant clinical interactions between Aripiprazole and alcohol/other medications are shown in Table 4.7.

Table 4.7 Most relevant clinical interactions between Aripiprazole and alcohol/other medications

Agent	Effect
Alcohol	Concomitant administration of Aripiprazole and alcohol may increase the risk of central nervous system depression.
Anti-hypertensive medications	Aripiprazole may increase their effects.
Carbamazepine and possibly other CYP450 3A4 inducers (e.g. barbiturates,	Concomitant administration of Aripiprazole and CYP450 3A4 inducers may result in

Table 4.7 (cont.)

Agent	Effect
Dexamethasone, Phenytoin, Rifampin, St John's wort)	lowered Aripiprazole levels: it may be appropriate to increase the dose of Aripiprazole.
Ketoconazole and possibly other CYP450 3A4 inhibitors (e.g. Aprepitant, azole anti-fungals, Fluoxetine, Fluvoxamine, grapefruit juice, macrolides, Nefazodone, protease inhibitors, Verapamil)	Concomitant administration of Aripiprazole and CYP450 3A4 inhibitors may result in raised Aripiprazole levels: it may be appropriate to decrease the dose of Aripiprazole.
Levodopa and dopamine-agonists	Aripiprazole may decrease their effects.
Quinidine and possibly other CYP450 2D6 inhibitors (e.g. Bupropion, Duloxetine, Fluoxetine, Paroxetine, Ritonavir, Sertraline)	Concomitant administration of Aripiprazole and CYP450 2D6 inhibitors may result in raised Aripiprazole levels: it may be appropriate to decrease the dose of Aripiprazole.

Special Populations

The main recommendations for the use of Aripiprazole in patients with hepatic and renal impairment are shown in Table 4.8.

Table 4.8 Main recommendations for the use of Aripiprazole in patients with hepatic and renal impairment

Hepatic impairment	Dose adjustment is not necessary.
Renal impairment	Dose adjustment is not necessary.

The main recommendations for the use of Aripiprazole during pregnancy and breast-feeding are shown in Table 4.9.

Table 4.9 Main recommendations for the use of Aripiprazole during pregnancy and breastfeeding

Pregnancy	Animal reproduction studies have shown adverse effects on the foetus and there are no controlled studies in humans, but potential benefits may warrant use of the medication in pregnant women despite potential risks. Overall, there is a risk of abnormal movements and withdrawal symptoms (agitation, hyper/hypotonia, tremor, sedation, breathing and/or feeding problems) in newborns whose mothers took an anti-dopaminergic medication during the third semester (former FDA Pregnancy Category C).
Breastfeeding	Evidence of excretion of Aripiprazole into breast milk: infants of women who choose to breastfeed while on Aripiprazole should be monitored for possible adverse effects.

Behavioural Neurology

Based on its particular mechanism of action (dopamine receptor partial agonism instead of antagonism), Aripiprazole is sometimes classed as a third generation anti-dopaminergic medication. Aripiprazole is also characterized by an overall better tolerability profile than most other anti-dopaminergic medications in terms of sedation, dyslipidaemia, diabetes mellitus, and weight gain (especially in adults). Aripiprazole does not affect blood pressure to the same extent as other anti-dopaminergic agents and therefore blood pressure monitoring is not mandatory for this medication. The same applies to other investigations, including electroencephalography. It has also been observed that low-dose Aripiprazole as adjunctive treatment can reverse the hyperprolactinaemia caused by other anti-dopaminergic agents. Aripiprazole has been approved for the adjunct treatment for depression and has been shown to be useful as augmentation therapying patients with Tourette syndrome with co-morbid obsessive-compulsive disorder. The first reports about the efficacy of Aripiprazole in controlling tics date back to the first decade of the new millennium. The growing evidence about the tic-suppressing properties of this medication, together with its favourable tolerability profile, explain its popularity as first/second-line pharmacotherapy in Tourette syndrome.

Guidelines

The main recommendations for the use of Aripiprazole according to the clinical guidelines on the treatment of tics are shown in Table 4.10.

Table 4.10 Main recommendations for the use of Aripiprazole according to published guidelines on the treatment of tics

Country (year)	Recommendation about Aripiprazole	Population
EU (+UK) (2011)	Evidence Level C; included as third medication in survey of preferred choices	Children + adults
EU (+UK) (2012)[a]	Included as third medication in top three recommendations (children) and first medication in top three recommendations (adults)	Children + adults
Canada (2012)	Weak recommendation, low-quality evidence	Children + adults
US (2013)	Listed with comments on tolerability (no prolactin elevation) and reports of improvement in obsessive-compulsive disorder	Children
UK (2016)	Moderate certainty in the effect estimate (children) (downgraded because of suboptimal sample size)	Children
Japan (2019)[a]	Included as first choice	Children + adults
US (2019)	Moderate certainty in the effect estimate (children) (based on one Class I study)	Children + adults

[a] Expert survey and consensus.

Overall Rating

A summary of the efficacy and tolerability profiles of Aripiprazole in patients with Tourette syndrome is presented in Table 4.11.

Table 4.11 Summary of efficacy and tolerability profiles of Aripiprazole in patients with Tourette syndrome

Efficacy for tics	☺☺
Efficacy for behavioural problems	☺☺
Tolerability	☺☺

☺☺☺ = very good
☺☺ = good
☺ = acceptable

Olanzapine

Pharmacological Properties

The main pharmacodynamic and pharmacokinetic properties of Olanzapine (Figure 4.2) are summarized in Table 4.12.

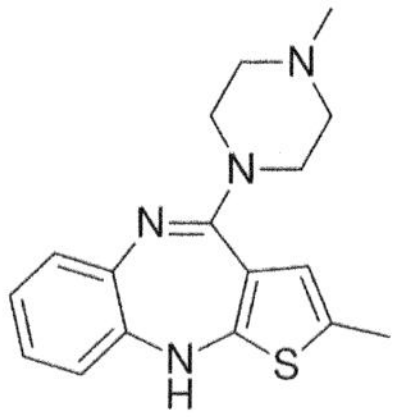

Figure 4.2 Olanzapine.

Table 4.12 Main pharmacodynamic and pharmacokinetic properties of Olanzapine

Mechanism(s) of action

Antagonism of D1, D2, D3, D4 dopamine receptors

Antagonism of 5-HT2A, 5-HT2B, 5-HT2C, 5-HT6 serotonin receptors

Antagonism of alpha-1 and alpha-2C adrenergic receptors

Antagonism of H1 histaminergic receptors

Antagonism of M1, M2, M3, M4 muscarinic cholinergic receptors

Pharmacokinetics

Peak effect in approximately 5–8 hours

Elimination half-life of approximately 40 hours

Eliminated in both urine and faeces (after extensive liver metabolism, mainly by CYP450 1A2 and CYP450 2D6)

Preparations

The relevant medicinal forms of Olanzapine are shown in Table 4.13.

Table 4.13 Relevant medicinal forms of Olanzapine

Tablets
Olanzapine 2.5 mg
Olanzapine 5 mg
Olanzapine 7.5 mg
Olanzapine 10 mg
Olanzapine 15 mg
Olanzapine 20 mg

Dose Titration

Dose is 2.5–5 mg daily for 14 days, then increased by 2.5–5 mg every 14 days; usual maintenance 5–20 mg once daily (maximum dose 20 mg daily).

Other Indications

The main clinical indications of Olanzapine in addition to tics are listed in Table 4.14.

Table 4.14 Main clinical indications of Olanzapine in addition to tics

Central nervous system conditions
Psychosis[a]
Bipolar affective disorder[a]
Treatment-refractory depression (in combination with Fluoxetine)[a]
Irritability and aggressiveness
Other conditions
–

[a] FDA approved.

Cautions

Caution is warranted when using Olanzapine in patients with the conditions listed in Table 4.15.

Adverse Effects

The overall tolerability of Olanzapine in terms of sedation and weight gain is shown in Table 4.16, whereas the frequency of individual adverse effects is presented in Table 4.17.

Table 4.15 Cautions about the use of Olanzapine

Central nervous system conditions

Central nervous system and respiratory depression

Other conditions

Angle-closure glaucoma, paralytic ileus, prostatic hypertrophy

Bone marrow depression, low leukocyte count, low neutrophil count

Conditions that predispose to hypotension (dehydration, overheating)

Hypereosinophilic disorders

Myeloproliferative disease

Table 4.16 Overall tolerability of Olanzapine in terms of sedation and weight gain

Sedation	☹☹
Weight gain	☹☹☹

☹☹☹ = significant problem
☹☹ = frequently reported
☹ = occasionally reported

Table 4.17 Frequency of adverse effects associated with Olanzapine

Very common (>1 in 10 patients on Olanzapine)	
CENTRAL NERVOUS SYSTEM: – Sedation	OTHER SYSTEMS: – Hyperprolactinaemia – Hypotension – Weight gain

Common (>1 in 100 patients on Olanzapine)	
CENTRAL NERVOUS SYSTEM: – Akathisia – Asthenia – Dizziness – Dyskinesias – Extrapyramidal symptoms – Fatigue – Somnolence	OTHER SYSTEMS: – Arthralgia – Constipation – Decreased libido – Dry mouth – Eosinophilia – Erectile dysfunction – Glycosuria – Hypercholesterolaemia – Hyperglycaemia – Hypertriglyceridaemia – Leukopenia – Liver enzyme abnormalities – Neutropenia

Table 4.17 (cont.)

Common (>1 in 100 patients on Olanzapine)

- Oedema
- Pyrexia
- Skin rash

Uncommon (>1 in 1000 patients on Olanzapine)

CENTRAL NERVOUS SYSTEM:

- Amnesia
- Dysarthria
- Dystonia
- Oculogyric crisis
- Restless legs syndrome
- Seizures

OTHER SYSTEMS:

- Abdominal distension
- Alopecia
- Amenorrhoea
- Bradycardia
- Diabetes mellitus
- Epistaxis
- Galactorrhoea
- Gynaecomastia
- Hyperbilirubinaemia
- Photosensitivity reaction
- QT prolongation
- Thromboembolism
- Urinary incontinence/retention

Rare (>1 in 10 000 patients on Olanzapine)

CENTRAL NERVOUS SYSTEM:

- Neuroleptic malignant syndrome

OTHER SYSTEMS:

- Hepatitis
- Hypothermia
- Pancreatitis
- Priapism
- Rhabdomyolysis
- Thrombocytopenia
- Ventricular tachycardia

Very rare (<1 in 10 000 patients on Olanzapine)

CENTRAL NERVOUS SYSTEM:

–

OTHER SYSTEMS:
– DRESS*

Abbreviations. DRESS, drug reaction with eosinophilia and systemic symptoms.

Interactions

The most relevant clinical interactions between Olanzapine and alcohol/other medications are shown in Table 4.18.

Special Populations

The main recommendations for the use of Olanzapine in patients with hepatic and renal impairment are shown in Table 4.19.

Table 4.18 Most relevant clinical interactions between Olanzapine and alcohol/other medications

Agent	Effect
Alcohol	Concomitant administration of Olanzapine and alcohol may increase the risk of central nervous system depression and hypotension.
Anti-hypertensive medications	Olanzapine may increase their effects.
Carbamazepine and other potent CYP450 1A2 inducers (e.g. cigarette smoke, Omeprazole, Rifampin)	Concomitant administration of Olanzapine and CYP450 1A2 inducers may result in lowered Olanzapine levels: it may be appropriate to increase the dose of Olanzapine.
Fluvoxamine and other potent CYP450 1A2 inhibitors (e.g. Fluoroquinolones, Verapamil)	Concomitant administration of Olanzapine and CYP450 1A2 inhibitors may result in raised Olanzapine levels: it may be appropriate to decrease the dose of Olanzapine.
Levodopa and dopamine-agonists	Olanzapine may decrease their effects.
Quinidine and possibly other potent CYP450 2D6 inhibitors (e.g. Bupropion, Fluoxetine, Paroxetine)	Concomitant administration of Olanzapine and CYP450 2D6 inhibitors may result in raised Olanzapine levels: it may be appropriate to decrease the dose of Olanzapine.

Table 4.19 Main recommendations for the use of Olanzapine in patients with hepatic and renal impairment

Hepatic impairment	Consider lower initial dose and increase with caution, especially in moderate to severe hepatic impairment.
Renal impairment	No dose adjustment is required for oral formulation.

The main recommendations for the use of Olanzapine during pregnancy and breast-feeding are shown in Table 4.20.

Table 4.20 Main recommendations for the use of Olanzapine during pregnancy and breastfeeding

Pregnancy	Animal reproduction studies have shown adverse effects on the foetus, and there are no controlled studies in humans, but potential benefits may warrant use of the medication in pregnant women despite potential risks. Overall, there is a risk of abnormal movements and withdrawal symptoms (agitation, hyper/hypotonia, tremor, sedation, breathing and/or feeding problems) in newborns whose mothers took an anti-dopaminergic medication during the third semester (former FDA Pregnancy Category C).
Breastfeeding	Evidence of excretion of Olanzapine into breast milk: infants of women who choose to breastfeed while on Olanzapine should be monitored for possible adverse effects.

Behavioural Neurology

In addition to its established use as anti-psychotic medication, Olanzapine is often used as a preferred augmenting agent in patients with bipolar affective disorder. Moreover, Olanzapine has documented efficacy as augmenting agent to Fluoxetine for treatment-refractory depression. Patients taking Olanzapine are mainly concerned about weight gain: obesity, diabetes mellitus and dyslipidaemia are among the most commonly reported adverse effects of this medication. Olanzapine has been shown to potentially have greater efficacy but also greater metabolic adverse effects compared to most first- and second-generation anti-dopaminergic medications (data from its use in patients with schizophrenia). There is some evidence for the efficacy of Olanzapine in the treatment of tics, especially in patients with Tourette syndrome and co-morbid obsessive-compulsive and affective symptoms. Tolerability issues limit its use also in patients with tics.

Guidelines

The main recommendations for the use of Olanzapine according to the clinical guidelines on the treatment of tics are shown in Table 4.21.

Table 4.21 Main recommendations for the use of Olanzapine according to published guidelines on the treatment of tics

Country (year)	Recommendation about Olanzapine	Population
EU (+UK) (2011)	Evidence Level B (with obsessive-compulsive behaviour as additional indication); not included in top three recommendations in survey of preferred choices	Children + adults
EU (+UK) (2012)[a]	Not included in top three recommendations	Children + adults
Canada (2012)	Weak recommendation, low-quality evidence	Children + adults
US (2013)	Listed with comments on adverse effects (metabolic effects as major concern)	Children
UK (2016)	Not listed	Children
Japan (2019)[a]	Not included as first/second choice	Children + adults
US (2019)	Not listed	Children + adults

[a] Expert survey and consensus.

Overall Rating

A summary of the efficacy and tolerability profiles of Olanzapine in patients with Tourette syndrome is presented in Table 4.22.

Table 4.22 Summary of efficacy and tolerability profiles of Olanzapine in patients with Tourette syndrome

Efficacy for tics	☺
Efficacy for behavioural problems	☺☺
Tolerability	☺

☺☺☺ = very good
☺☺ = good
☺ = acceptable

Quetiapine

Pharmacological Properties

The main pharmacodynamic and pharmacokinetic properties of Quetiapine (Figure 4.3) are summarized in Table 4.23.

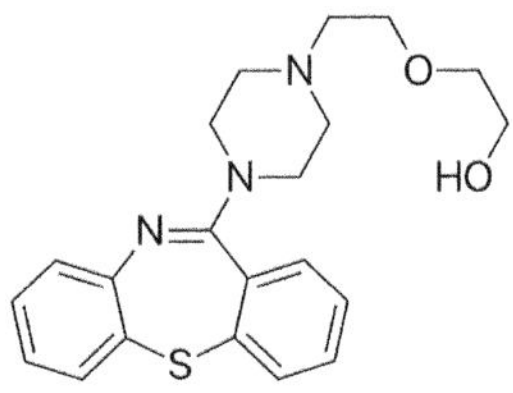

Figure 4.3 Quetiapine.

Table 4.23 Main pharmacodynamic and pharmacokinetic properties of Quetiapine

Mechanism(s) of action

Antagonism of D1[a], D2[a], D3[a] dopamine receptors

Partial agonism of 5-HT1A[a] serotonin receptors

Antagonism of 5-HT1D[a], 5-HT1E[a], 5-HT2A, 5-HT2B, 5-HT2C[a], 5-HT6[a], 5-HT7 serotonin receptors

Antagonism of alpha-1, alpha-2A[a], alpha-2B[a], alpha-2C[a] adrenergic receptors

Antagonism of H1 histaminergic receptors

Antagonism of M1, M2[a], M3, M4[a] muscarinic cholinergic receptors

Pharmacokinetics

Peak effect in approximately 1.5 hours (immediate release) or 6 hours (extended release)

Elimination half-life of approximately 6 hours

Eliminated in both urine and faeces (after extensive liver metabolism, mainly by CYP450 3A4)

[a] At higher doses.

Preparations

The relevant medicinal forms of Quetiapine are shown in Table 4.24.

Dose Titration

Immediate release. Dose is 25–50 mg daily for 14 days, then increased by 50 mg every 14 days; usual maintenance 300–600 mg daily in two divided doses (maximum dose 800 mg daily).

Table 4.24 Relevant medicinal forms of Quetiapine

Tablets

Quetiapine 25 mg (immediate release)

Quetiapine 50 mg (immediate release)

Quetiapine 100 mg (immediate release)

Quetiapine 200 mg (immediate release)

Quetiapine 300 mg (immediate release)

Quetiapine 50 mg (extended release)

Quetiapine 150 mg (extended release)

Quetiapine 200 mg (extended release)

Quetiapine 300 mg (extended release)

Quetiapine 400 mg (extended release)

Oral suspension

Quetiapine 20 mg/1 ml

Extended release. Dose is 50 mg daily for 14 days, then increased by 50 mg every 14 days; usual maintenance 300–600 mg once daily (maximum dose 800 mg daily).

Other Indications

The main clinical indications of Quetiapine in addition to tics are listed in Table 4.25.

Table 4.25 Main clinical indications of Quetiapine in addition to tics

Central nervous system conditions

Psychosis[a]

Bipolar affective disorder[a]

Depression (adjunctive therapy)[a]

Irritability and aggressiveness

Obsessive-compulsive disorder (augmentation therapy)

Anxiety

Other conditions

–

[a] FDA approved.

Cautions

Caution is warranted when using Quetiapine in patients with the conditions listed in Table 4.26.

Table 4.26 Cautions about the use of Quetiapine

Central nervous system conditions

Cerebrovascular disease

Other conditions

Cardiovascular disease

Conditions that predispose to hypotension (dehydration, overheating)

Elderly and patients at risk of aspiration pneumonia[a]

[a] Potentially caused by dysphagia.

Adverse Effects

The overall tolerability of Quetiapine in terms of sedation and weight gain is shown in Table 4.27, whereas the frequency of individual adverse effects is presented in Table 4.28.

Table 4.27 Overall tolerability of Quetiapine in terms of sedation and weight gain

Sedation	☹☹☹
Weight gain	☹☹

☹☹☹ = significant problem
☹☹ = frequently reported
☹ = occasionally reported

Table 4.28 Frequency of adverse effects associated with Quetiapine

Very common (>1 in 10 patients on Quetiapine)	
CENTRAL NERVOUS SYSTEM:	OTHER SYSTEMS:
– Dizziness	– Dry mouth
– Extrapyramidal symptoms	– Haemoglobin decrease
– Headache	– Hypertrygliceridaemia
– Sedation	– Hypercholesterolaemia
	– Weight gain
Common (>1 in 100 patients on Quetiapine)	
CENTRAL NERVOUS SYSTEM:	OTHER SYSTEMS:
– Asthenia	– Blurred vision
– Dysarthria	– Constipation

Table 4.28 (cont.)

Common (>1 in 100 patients on Quetiapine)

- Irritability
- Nightmares
- Suicidal ideation/behaviour[a]

- Dyspepsia
- Dyspnoea
- Eosinophilia
- Hyperglycaemia
- Hyperprolactinaemia
- Hypotension
- Increased appetite
- Leukopenia
- Liver enzyme abnormalities
- Nausea and vomiting
- Oedema
- Palpitations
- Pyrexia
- Tachycardia
- Thyroid function abnormalities

Uncommon (>1 in 1000 patients on Quetiapine)

CENTRAL NERVOUS SYSTEM:

- Restless legs syndrome
- Seizures
- Tardive dyskinesias

OTHER SYSTEMS:

- Anaemia
- Bradycardia
- Diabetes mellitus
- Dysphagia
- Hyponatraemia
- Hypothyroidism
- Neutropenia
- QT prolongation
- Rhinitis
- Sexual dysfunction
- Skin reactions
- Syncope
- Thrombocytopenia
- Urinary retention

Rare (>1 in 10 000 patients on Quetiapine)

CENTRAL NERVOUS SYSTEM:

- Neuroleptic malignant syndrome
- Somnambulism, sleep talking, sleep related eating disorder

OTHER SYSTEMS:

- Agranulocytosis
- Galactorrhoea
- Gynaecomastia
- Hepatitis
- Hypothermia
- Intestinal obstruction
- Jaundice
- Menstrual disorder
- Metabolic syndrome

Table 4.28 (cont.)

Rare (>1 in 10 000 patients on Quetiapine)

- Pancreatitis
- Priapism
- Thromboembolism

Very rare (<1 in 10 000 patients on Quetiapine)

CENTRAL NERVOUS SYSTEM:	OTHER SYSTEMS:
–	– Anaphylactic reaction
	– Angioedema
	– Inappropriate anti-diuretic hormone secretion
	– Rhabdomyolisis
	– Stevens–Johnson syndrome

[a] Particularly on initiation.

Interactions

The most relevant clinical interactions between Quetiapine and alcohol/other medications are shown in Table 4.29.

Table 4.29 Most relevant clinical interactions between Quetiapine and alcohol/other medications

Agent	Effect
Alcohol	Concomitant administration of Quetiapine and alcohol may increase the risk of central nervous system depression and hypotension.
Carbamazepine and possibly other CYP450 3A4 inducers (e.g. barbiturates, Dexamethasone, Phenytoin, Rifampin, St John's wort)	Concomitant administration of Quetiapine and CYP450 3A4 inducers may result in lowered Quetiapine levels: it may be appropriate to increase the dose of Quetiapine.
Ketoconazole and possibly other CYP450 3A4 inhibitors (e.g. Aprepitant, azole anti-fungals, Fluoxetine, Fluvoxamine, grapefruit juice, macrolides, Nefazodone, protease inhibitors, Verapamil)	Concomitant administration of Quetiapine and CYP450 3A4 inhibitors may result in raised Quetiapine levels: it may be appropriate to decrease the dose of Quetiapine.
Lorazepam	Quetiapine may slightly decrease its levels.
Quinidine and possibly other potent CYP450 2D6 inhibitors (e.g. Bupropion, Fluoxetine, Paroxetine)	Concomitant administration of Quetiapine and CYP450 2D6 inhibitors may result in raised Quetiapine levels; however, dosage reduction of Quetiapine is not usually necessary.
Valproate	Quetiapine may slightly decrease its levels.
Warfarin	There are case reports of increased International Normalized Ratio when Quetiapine is co-administered with Warfarin (also a substrate of CYP450 3A4).

Special Populations

The main recommendations for the use of Quetiapine in patients with hepatic and renal impairment are shown in Table 4.30.

Table 4.30 Main recommendations for the use of Quetiapine in patients with hepatic and renal impairment

Hepatic impairment	Consider lower initial dose and increase with caution.
Renal impairment	No dose adjustment is required for oral formulation.

The main recommendations for the use of Quetiapine during pregnancy and breastfeeding are shown in Table 4.31.

Table 4.31 Main recommendations for the use of Quetiapine during pregnancy and breastfeeding

Pregnancy	Animal reproduction studies have shown adverse effects on the foetus, and there are no controlled studies in humans, but potential benefits may warrant use of the medication in pregnant women despite potential risks. Overall, there is a risk of abnormal movements and withdrawal symptoms (agitation, hyper/hypotonia, tremor, sedation, breathing and/or feeding problems) in newborns whose mothers took an anti-dopaminergic medication during the third semester (former FDA Pregnancy Category C).
Breastfeeding	Evidence of excretion of Quetiapine into breast milk: infants of women who choose to breastfeed while on Quetiapine should be monitored for possible adverse effects.

Behavioural Neurology

At pharmacodynamic level, Quetiapine exerts different effects depending on the dose: higher doses usually achieve greater response for psychotic or manic symptoms, whereas lower doses can be effective for the treatment of anxiety and affective symptoms. Sedation is the most clinically relevant adverse effect, as hyperprolactinaemia and motor adverse effects are less severe compared to other anti-dopaminergic agents. Quetiapine is the preferred anti-dopaminergic medication for the treatment of iatrogenic psychosis and impulse control disorders in patients with Parkinson disease. There is limited evidence for the efficacy of Quetiapine for the treatment of tics, especially in comparison to other anti-dopaminergic medications.

Guidelines

The main recommendations for the use of Quetiapine according to the clinical guidelines on the treatment of tics are shown in Table 4.32.

Overall Rating

A summary of the efficacy and tolerability profiles of Quetiapine in patients with Tourette syndrome is presented in Table 4.33.

Table 4.32 Main recommendations for the use of Quetiapine according to published guidelines on the treatment of tics

Country (year)	Recommendation about Quetiapine	Population
EU (+UK) (2011)	Evidence Level C; included as tenth medication in survey of preferred choices	Children + adults
EU (+UK) (2012)[a]	[not included in top three recommendations]	Children + adults
Canada (2012)	Weak recommendatio; very low quality evidence	Children + adults
US (2013)	Listed with comments on adverse effects (metabolic effects)	Children
UK (2016)	[not listed]	Children
Japan (2019)[a]	[not included as first/second choice]	Children + adults
US (2019)	[not listed]	Children + adults

[a] Expert survey and consensus.

Table 4.33 Summary of efficacy and tolerability profiles of Quetiapine in patients with Tourette syndrome

Efficacy for tics	☺
Efficacy for behavioural problems	☺☺
Tolerability	☺☺

☺☺☺ = very good
☺☺ = good
☺ = acceptable

Risperidone

Pharmacological Properties

The main pharmacodynamic and pharmacokinetic properties of Risperidone (Figure 4.4) are summarized in Table 4.34.

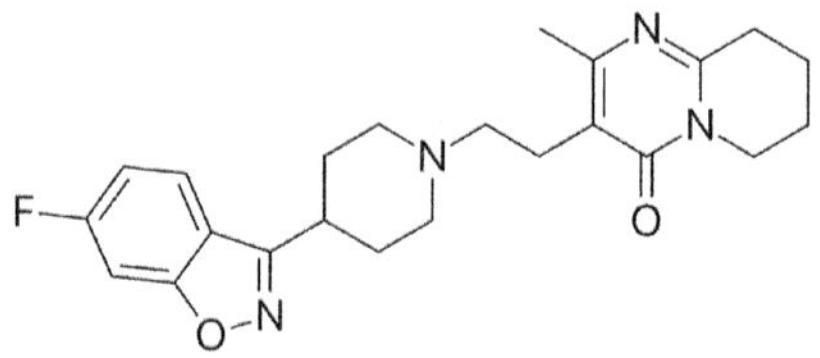

Figure 4.4 Risperidone.

Table 4.34 Main pharmacodynamic and pharmacokinetic properties of Risperidone

Mechanism(s) of action

Antagonism of D2, D3, D4 dopamine receptors

Antagonism of 5-HT1B, 5-HT1D, 5-HT2A, 5-HT2B, 5-HT2C, 5-HT7 serotonin receptors

Antagonism of alpha-1, alpha-2A, alpha-2B, alpha-2C adrenergic receptors

Antagonism of H1 histaminergic receptors

Pharmacokinetics

Peak effect in approximately 1–2 hours

Elimination half-life of approximately 22 hours

Eliminated mainly in urine (after extensive liver metabolism, mainly by CYP450 2D6)

Preparations

The relevant medicinal forms of Risperidone are shown in Table 4.35.

Table 4.35 Relevant medicinal forms of Risperidone

Tablets

Risperidone 0.5 mg

Risperidone 1 mg

Risperidone 2 mg

Risperidone 3 mg

Risperidone 4 mg

Risperidone 6 mg

Oral solution

Risperidone 1 mg/1 ml

Dose Titration

Dose is 0.5–1 mg daily for 14 days, then increased by 0.5–1 mg every 14 days; usual maintenance 1–6 mg daily in one to two divided doses (maximum dose 16 mg daily).

Other Indications

The main clinical indications of Risperidone in addition to tics are listed in Table 4.36.

Cautions

Caution is warranted when using Risperidone in patients with the conditions listed in Table 4.37.

Table 4.36 Main clinical indications of Risperidone in addition to tics

Central nervous system conditions

Psychosis[a]

Bipolar affective disorder[a]

Irritability and aggressiveness

Obsessive-compulsive disorder (augmentation therapy)

Other conditions

–

[a] FDA approved.

Table 4.37 Cautions about the use of Risperidone

Central nervous system conditions

Parkinson disease, Lewy body dementia

Other conditions

Acute porphyrias[a]

Cardiovascular disease

Cataract surgery

Conditions that predispose to hypotension (dehydration, overheating)

Elderly and patients at risk of aspiration pneumonia[b]

Prolactin-dependent tumours

[a] Contraindication. [b] Potentially caused by dysphagia.

Adverse Effects

The overall tolerability of Risperidone in terms of sedation and weight gain is shown in Table 4.38, whereas the frequency of individual adverse effects is presented in Table 4.39.

Table 4.38 Overall tolerability of Risperidone in terms of sedation and weight gain

Sedation	☹☹
Weight gain	☹☹

☹☹☹ = significant problem
☹☹ = frequently reported
☹ = occasionally reported

Table 4.39 Frequency of adverse effects associated with Risperidone

Very common (>1 in 10 patients on Risperidone)

CENTRAL NERVOUS SYSTEM:

- Extrapyramidal symptoms
- Headache
- Insomnia
- Sedation

OTHER SYSTEMS:

-

Common (>1 in 100 patients on Risperidone)

CENTRAL NERVOUS SYSTEM:

- Agitation
- Akathisia
- Anxiety
- Asthenia
- Depression
- Dizziness
- Dyskinesias
- Dystonia
- Fatigue
- Pain
- Sleep disorders
- Tremor

OTHER SYSTEMS:

- Abdominal pain/discomfort
- Appetite changes
- Arthralgia
- Blurred vision
- Chest pain
- Conjunctivitis
- Constipation
- Cough
- Diarrhoea
- Dry mouth
- Dyspepsia
- Dyspnoea
- Epistaxis, nasal congestion
- Erythema
- Hyperprolactinaemia
- Hypertension
- Muscle spasms/pain
- Nausea and vomiting
- Oedema
- Pyrexia
- Respiratory/urinary tract infections
- Skin rash
- Tachycardia
- Urinary incontinence
- Weight gain

Uncommon (>1 in 1000 patients on Risperidone)

CENTRAL NERVOUS SYSTEM:

- Ataxia
- Attentional deficit
- Central nervous system depression
- Confusion
- Decreased libido
- Dysgeusia

OTHER SYSTEMS:

- Alopecia
- Amenorrhoea
- Anaemia
- Anorexia
- Atrial fibrillation
- Bradycardia
- Diabetes mellitus

Table 4.39 (cont.)

Uncommon (>1 in 1000 patients on Risperidone)

- Hyperactivity
- Irritability
- Mania
- Nightmares
- Paraesthesias, hypoaesthesia
- Seizures
- Tardive dyskinesias
- Thirst

- Dry eyes
- Dysphagia
- Dysphonia
- Erectile dysfunction
- Eosinophilia
- Flatulence
- Galactorrhoea
- Gynaecomastia
- Gastroenteritis
- Hypercholesterolaemia
- Hyperglycaemia
- Hyperthermia
- Hypotension
- Increased lacrimation
- Leukopenia
- Liver enzyme abnormalities
- Muscle stiffness/weakness
- Neutropenia
- Palpitations
- Polydipsia
- Pruritus
- QT prolongation
- Respiratory disorders
- Skin reactions
- Syncope
- Thrombocytopenia
- Tinnitus
- Urinary retention, dysuria
- Vertigo, tinnitus, ear pain

Rare (>1 in 10 000 patients on Risperidone)

CENTRAL NERVOUS SYSTEM:

- Anorgasmia
- Catatonia
- Cerebrovascular disorder
- Neuroleptic malignant syndrome
- Somnambulism, sleep related eating disorder

OTHER SYSTEMS:

- Agranulocytosis
- Anaphylactic reaction
- Eye movement disorders
- Glaucoma
- Glucosuria
- Hyperinsulinaemia
- Hypertrygliceridaemia
- Hypoglycaemia
- Hypothermia
- Inappropriate anti-diuretic hormone secretion
- Intestinal obstruction

Table 4.39 (cont.)

Rare (>1 in 10 000 patients on Risperidone)
– Jaundice
– Menstrual disorder
– Pancreatitis
– Priapism
– Rhabdomyolysis
– Sinus arrhythmia
– Sleep apnoea syndrome
– Thromboembolism

Very rare (<1 in 10 000 patients on Risperidone)	
CENTRAL NERVOUS SYSTEM:	OTHER SYSTEMS:
–	– Angioedema
	– Diabetic ketoacidosis

Interactions

The most relevant clinical interactions between Risperidone and alcohol/other medications are shown in Table 4.40.

Table 4.40 Most relevant clinical interactions between Risperidone and alcohol/other medications

Agent	Effect
Alcohol	Concomitant administration of Risperidone and alcohol may increase the risk of central nervous system depression.
Anti-hypertensive medications	Risperidone may increase their effects.
Carbamazepine	Concomitant administration of Risperidone and Carbamazepine may result in lowered Risperidone levels.
Clozapine	Concomitant administration of Risperidone and Clozapine may result in raised Risperidone levels because of its reduced clearance; however, dosage reduction of Risperidone is not usually necessary.
Levodopa and dopamine-agonists	Risperidone may decrease their effects.
Quinidine and possibly other potent CYP450 2D6 inhibitors (e.g. Bupropion, Fluoxetine, Paroxetine)	Concomitant administration of Risperidone and CYP450 2D6 inhibitors may result in raised Risperidone levels; however, dosage reduction of Risperidone is not usually necessary.

Special Populations

The main recommendations for the use of Risperidone in patients with hepatic and renal impairment are shown in Table 4.41.

Table 4.41 Main recommendations for the use of Risperidone in patients with hepatic and renal impairment

Hepatic impairment	Initial and subsequent oral doses should be halved.
Renal impairment	Initial and subsequent oral doses should be halved.

The main recommendations for the use of Risperidone during pregnancy and breastfeeding are shown in Table 4.42.

Table 4.42 Main recommendations for the use of Risperidone during pregnancy and breastfeeding

Pregnancy	Animal reproduction studies have shown adverse effects on the foetus and there are no controlled studies in humans, but potential benefits may warrant use of the medication in pregnant women despite potential risks. Overall, there is a risk of abnormal movements and withdrawal symptoms (agitation, hyper/hypotonia, tremor, sedation, breathing and/or feeding problems) in newborns whose mothers took an anti-dopaminergic medication during the third semester (former FDA Pregnancy Category C).
Breastfeeding	Evidence of excretion of Risperidone into breast milk: infants of women who choose to breastfeed while on Risperidone should be monitored for possible adverse effects.

Behavioural Neurology

Among second-generation anti-dopaminergic medications, Risperidone was the first agent to be identified as a powerful treatment for tics, as well as psychosis. Compared to first-generation anti-dopaminergic medications, Risperidone and the other second-generation anti-dopaminergic agents are characterized by a better tolerability profile in terms of extrapyramidal symptoms and tardive dyskinesias, although the metabolic adverse effects can be clinically relevant. In addition to its known anti-tic effects, Risperidone has been shown to be an effective medication for the augmentation therapy of co-morbid obsessive-compulsive disorder in patients with Tourette syndrome. Tolerability can still be an issue (e.g. dose-dependent hyperprolactinaemia); sedation and weight gain have been shown to potentially affect general health particularly in younger patients.

Guidelines

The main recommendations for the use of Risperidone according to the clinical guidelines on the treatment of tics are shown in Table 4.43.

Table 4.43 Main recommendations for the use of Risperidone according to published guidelines on the treatment of tics

Country (year)	Recommendation about Risperidone	Population
EU (+UK) (2011)	Evidence Level A (with disruptive behaviour disorder as additional indication); included as first medication in survey of preferred choices	Children + adults
EU (+UK) (2012)[a]	Included as first medication in top three recommendations (children) and second medication in top three recommendations (adults)	Children + adults

Table 4.43 (cont.)

Country (year)	Recommendation about Risperidone	Population
Canada (2012)	Weak recommendation, high-quality evidence	Children + adults
US (2013)	Listed with comments on adverse effects (metabolic effects, prolactin elevation)	Children
UK (2016)	Low certainty in the effect estimate (children) (downgraded because of suboptimal sample size)	Children
Japan (2019)[a]	Included as both first and second choice	Children + adults
US (2019)	Moderate certainty in the effect estimate (children + adults) (based on two Class II studies)	Children + adults

[a] Expert survey and consensus.

Overall Rating

A summary of the efficacy and tolerability profiles of Risperidone in patients with Tourette syndrome is presented in Table 4.44.

Table 4.44 Summary of efficacy and tolerability profiles of Risperidone in patients with Tourette syndrome

Efficacy for tics	☺☺☺
Efficacy for behavioural problems	☺☺
Tolerability	☺

☺☺☺ = very good
☺☺ = good
☺ = acceptable

Ziprasidone

The main pharmacodynamic and pharmacokinetic properties of Ziprasidone (Figure 4.5) are summarized in Table 4.45.

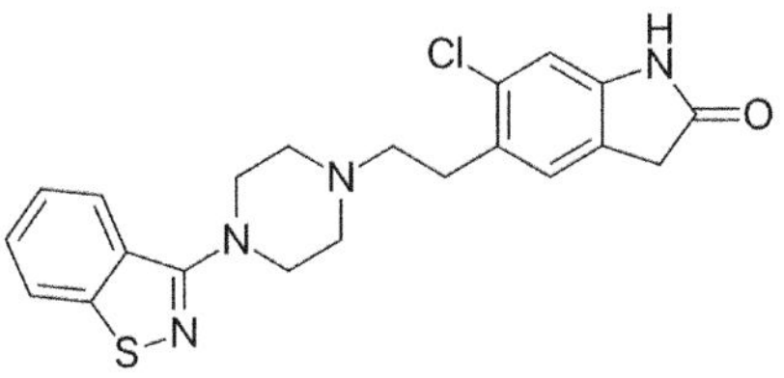

Figure 4.5 Ziprasidone.

Table 4.45 Main pharmacodynamic and pharmacokinetic properties of Ziprasidone

Mechanism(s) of action

Antagonism of D2 and D3 dopamine receptors

Partial agonism of 5-HT1A serotonin receptors

Antagonism of 5-HT1B, 5-HT1D, 5-HT2A, 5-HT2B, 5-HT2C, 5-HT6, 5-HT7 serotonin receptors

Antagonism of alpha-1, alpha-2B, alpha-2C adrenergic receptors

Antagonism of NET (norepinephrine transporter)

Antagonism of H1 histaminergic receptors

Pharmacokinetics

Peak effect in approximately 6–8 hours

Elimination half-life of approximately 7 hours

Eliminated mainly in the faeces (after extensive liver metabolism, mainly by CYP450 3A4)

Preparations

The relevant medicinal forms of Ziprasidone are shown in Table 4.46.

Table 4.46 Relevant medicinal forms of Ziprasidone

Capsules
Ziprasidone 20 mg
Ziprasidone 40 mg
Ziprasidone 60 mg
Ziprasidone 80 mg

Dose Titration

Dose is 20 mg daily for 14 days, then increased by 20 mg every 14 days; usual maintenance 20–60 mg daily in one to two divided doses (maximum dose 200 mg daily).

Other Indications

The main clinical indications of Ziprasidone in addition to tics are listed in Table 4.47.

Cautions

Caution is warranted when using Ziprasidone in patients with the conditions listed in Table 4.48.

Adverse Effects

The overall tolerability of Ziprasidone in terms of sedation and weight gain is shown in Table 4.49, whereas the frequency of individual adverse effects is presented in Table 4.50.

Table 4.47 Main clinical indications of Ziprasidone in addition to tics

Central nervous system conditions

Psychosis[a]

Bipolar affective disorder[a]

Irritability and aggressiveness

Other conditions

–

[a] FDA approved.

Table 4.48 Cautions about the use of Ziprasidone

Central nervous system conditions

–

Other conditions

History of arrhythmias[a], recent acute myocardial infarction[a], uncompensated heart failure[a], history or family history of congenital QT prolongation[a], co-administration of medications capable of prolonging the QT interval (e.g. selected anti-arrhythmics, Moxifloxacine, Pimozide, Sparfloxacin, Thioridazine)[a]

Conditions that predispose to hypotension (dehydration, overheating)

Elderly and patients at risk of aspiration pneumonia[b]

[a] Contraindication. [b]Potentially caused by dysphagia.

Table 4.49 Overall tolerability of Ziprasidone in terms of sedation and weight gain

Sedation	☹
Weight gain	☹

☹☹☹ = significant problem
☹☹ = frequently reported
☹ = occasionally reported

Interactions

The most relevant clinical interactions between Ziprasidone and alcohol/other medications are shown in Table 4.51.

Special Populations

The main recommendations for the use of Ziprasidone in patients with hepatic and renal impairment are shown in Table 4.52.

Table 4.50 Frequency of adverse effects associated with Ziprasidone

Very common (>1 in 10 patients on Ziprasidone)

CENTRAL NERVOUS SYSTEM:
- Headache
- Insomnia
- Sedation

OTHER SYSTEMS:
-

Common (>1 in 100 patients on Ziprasidone)

CENTRAL NERVOUS SYSTEM:
- Agitation
- Akathisia
- Anxiety
- Asthenia
- Dizziness
- Dyskinesias
- Dystonia
- Extrapyramidal symptoms
- Fatigue
- Hypertonia
- Mania
- Pain
- Restlessness
- Tardive dyskinesias
- Tremor

OTHER SYSTEMS:
- Blurred vision
- Constipation
- Dry eye
- Dry mouth
- Dyspepsia
- Hypersalivation
- Hypertension
- Muscle stiffness
- Nausea and vomiting
- Pyrexia
- Rhinitis
- Skin rash
- Tachycardia
- Weight changes

Uncommon (>1 in 1000 patients on Ziprasidone)

CENTRAL NERVOUS SYSTEM:
- Akinesia
- Ataxia
- Attentional deficit
- Central nervous system depression
- Decreased libido
- Depression
- Dysarthria
- Irritability
- Nightmares
- Oculogyric crisis
- Panic attacks
- Paraesthesias, hypoaesthesia
- Restless legs syndrome
- Seizures
- Thirst

OTHER SYSTEMS:
- Alopecia
- Amenorrhoea
- Dysphagia
- Dyspnoea
- Flatulence
- Galactorrhoea
- Gastritis
- Gynaecomastia
- Hypotension
- Liver enzyme abnormalities
- Muscle spasms/pain
- Palpitations
- QT prolongation
- Skin reactions
- Syncope
- Urinary incontinence, dysuria
- Vertigo, tinnitus, ear pain

Rare (>1 in 10 000 patients on Ziprasidone)	
CENTRAL NERVOUS SYSTEM:	OTHER SYSTEMS:
– Anorgasmia	– Amblyopia
– Ataxia	– Angioedema
– Facial droop	– DRESS*
– Paresis	– Erectile dysfunction
– Hypomania	– Hiccups
– Neuroleptic malignant syndrome	– Hyperprolactinaemia
– Serotonin syndrome	– Increased appetite
	– Laryngospasm
	– Priapism
	– Psoriasis
	– Torsade de pointes
	– Urinary retention, enuresis
Very rare (<1 in 10 000 patients on Ziprasidone)	
CENTRAL NERVOUS SYSTEM:	OTHER SYSTEMS:
–	– Anaphylactic reaction
	– Embolism
	– Eosinophilia
	– Lymphopenia

Abbreviations. DRESS, drug reaction with eosinophilia and systemic symptoms.

Table 4.51 Most relevant clinical interactions between Ziprasidone and alcohol/other medications

Agent	Effect
Alcohol	Concomitant administration of Ziprasidone and alcohol may increase the risk of central nervous system depression.
Anti-hypertensive medications	Ziprasidone may increase their effects.
Levodopa and dopamine-agonists	Ziprasidone may decrease their effects.
Medications capable of prolonging the QT interval (e.g. selected anti-arrhythmics, Moxifloxacine, Pimozide, Sparfloxacin, Thioridazine)	Concomitant administration of Ziprasidone and medications capable of significantly prolonging the QT interval may increase the risk of arrhythmias.

The main recommendations for the use of Ziprasidone during pregnancy and breast-feeding are shown in Table 4.53.

Table 4.52 Main recommendations for the use of Ziprasidone in patients with hepatic and renal impairment

Hepatic impairment	No dose adjustment is necessary.
Renal impairment	No dose adjustment is necessary.

Table 4.53 Main recommendations for the use of Ziprasidone during pregnancy and breastfeeding

Pregnancy	Animal reproduction studies have shown adverse effects on the foetus and there are no controlled studies in humans, but potential benefits may warrant use of the medication in pregnant women despite potential risks. Overall, there is a risk of abnormal movements and withdrawal symptoms (agitation, hyper/hypotonia, tremor, sedation, breathing and/or feeding problems) in newborns whose mothers took an anti-dopaminergic medication during the third semester (former FDA Pregnancy Category C).
Breastfeeding	Evidence of excretion of Ziprasidone into breast milk: infants of women who choose to breastfeed while on Ziprasidone should be monitored for possible adverse effects.

Behavioural Neurology

Ziprasidone is mainly used to treat patients with forms of psychosis and bipolar affective disorder that are refractory to other anti-dopaminergic medications. As with the first-generation anti-dopaminergic agent Pimozide, Ziprasidone carries a risk of QT prolongation, which can become clinically significant if patients are prescribed medications that have the potential to increase the plasma level of Ziprasidone. There is some evidence that Ziprasidone has less severe metabolic adverse effects than other anti-dopaminergic medications. The risk of developing diabetes mellitus, dyslipidaemia and weight gain appears to be lower with Ziprasidone. With regard to its use for the treatment of tics, the available evidence is mainly based on trials with doses that are substantially inferior to the doses of the currently available formulations.

Guidelines

The main recommendations for the use of Ziprasidone according to the clinical guidelines on the treatment of tics are shown in Table 4.54.

Table 4.54 Main recommendations for the use of Ziprasidone according to published guidelines on the treatment of tics

Country (year)	Recommendation about Ziprasidone	Population
EU (+UK) (2011)	Evidence Level A; included as ninth medication in survey of preferred choices	Children + adults
EU (+UK) (2012)[a]	Not included in top three recommendations	Children + adults
Canada (2012)	Weak recommendation, low-quality evidence (children)	Children + adults
US (2013)		Children

Table 4.54 (cont.)

Country (year)	Recommendation about Ziprasidone	Population
	Listed with comments on current available doses being above those used in randomized controlled trials	
UK (2016)	Low certainty in the effect estimate (children) (downgraded because of suboptimal sample size and high risk of bias)	Children
Japan (2019)[a]	Not included as first/second choice	Children + adults
US (2019)	Low certainty in the effect estimate (children) (based on one Class II study)	Children + adults

[a] Expert survey and consensus.

Overall Rating

A summary of the efficacy and tolerability profiles of Ziprasidone in patients with Tourette syndrome is presented in Table 4.55.

Table 4.55 Summary of efficacy and tolerability profiles of Ziprasidone in patients with Tourette syndrome

Efficacy for tics	☺☺
Efficacy for behavioural problems	☺
Tolerability	☺

☺☺☺ = very good
☺☺ = good
☺ = acceptable

Alpha-2 Adrenergic Medications

Clonidine

Pharmacological Properties

The main pharmacodynamic and pharmacokinetic properties of Clonidine (Figure 5.1) are summarized in Table 5.1.

Figure 5.1 Clonidine.

Table 5.1 Main pharmacodynamic and pharmacokinetic properties of Clonidine

Mechanism(s) of action

Agonism of alpha-2A adrenergic receptors (lower affinity for alpha-2B and alpha-2C adrenergic receptors)

Pharmacokinetics

Peak effect in approximately 2–4 hours

Elimination half-life of approximately 14 hours

Eliminated in urine following hepatic metabolism

Preparations

The relevant medicinal forms of Clonidine are shown in Table 5.2.

Table 5.2 Relevant medicinal forms of Clonidine

Tablets

Clonidine 0.025 mg

Clonidine 0.1 mg

Oral solution

Clonidine 0.05 mg/5 ml

Dose Titration

Dose is 0.025 mg daily for 14 days, then increased by 0.025 mg every 14 days; usual maintenance 0.1–0.4 mg daily in two to three divided doses (maximum dose 1.2 mg daily).

Other Indications

The main clinical indications of Clonidine in addition to tics are listed in Table 5.3.

Table 5.3 Main clinical indications of Clonidine in addition to tics

Central nervous system conditions

Attention-deficit and hyperactivity disorder[a]

Irritability and aggressiveness

Anxiety

Alcohol and opiate withdrawal syndrome

Other conditions

Hypertension[a]

Neuropathic pain

Hyperhidrosis

[a] FDA approved.

Cautions

Caution is warranted when using Clonidine in patients with the conditions listed in Table 5.4.

Table 5.4 Cautions about the use of Clonidine

Central nervous system conditions

History of depression

Other conditions

Bradyarrhythmia (mild to moderate)

Bradyarrhythmia (severe) secondary to atrio-ventricular block or sick sinus syndrome[a]

Cerebrovascular disease

Constipation

Heart failure

Polyneuropathy

Raynaud phenomenon or other occlusive peripheral vascular disease

[a] Contraindication.

Adverse Effects

The overall tolerability of Clonidine in terms of sedation and weight gain is shown in Table 5.5, whereas the frequency of individual adverse effects is presented in Table 5.6.

Table 5.5 Overall tolerability of Clonidine in terms of sedation and weight gain

Sedation	☹☹
Weight gain	–

☹☹☹ = significant problem
☹☹ = frequently reported
☹ = occasionally reported

Table 5.6 Frequency of adverse effects associated with Clonidine

Very common (>1 in 10 patients on Clonidine)	
CENTRAL NERVOUS SYSTEM:	OTHER SYSTEMS:
– Dizziness	– Dry mouth
– Sedation	– Orthostatic hypotension

Common (>1 in 100 patients on Clonidine)	
CENTRAL NERVOUS SYSTEM:	OTHER SYSTEMS:
– Depression	– Constipation
– Fatigue	– Erectile dysfunction
– Headache	– Nausea and vomiting
– Sleep disorders	– Salivary gland pain

Uncommon (>1 in 1000 patients on Clonidine)	
CENTRAL NERVOUS SYSTEM:	OTHER SYSTEMS:
– Delusions	– Malaise
– Hallucinations	– Pruritus
– Nightmares	– Raynaud phenomenon
– Paraesthesias	– Sinus bradycardia
	– Skin rash
	– Urticaria

Rare (>1 in 10 000 patients on Clonidine)	
CENTRAL NERVOUS SYSTEM:	OTHER SYSTEMS:
–	– Alopecia
	– Atrio-ventricular block
	– Colonic pseudo-obstruction
	– Decreased lacrimation
	– Gynaecomastia
	– Hyperglycaemia
	– Nasal dryness

Very rare (<1 in 10 000 patients on Clonidine)	
CENTRAL NERVOUS SYSTEM:	OTHER SYSTEMS:
–	–

Interactions

The most relevant clinical interactions between Clonidine and alcohol/other medications are shown in Table 5.7.

Table 5.7 Most relevant clinical interactions between Clonidine and alcohol/other medications

Agent	Effect
Alcohol and central nervous system depressant agents	Concomitant administration of Clonidine and alcohol (or other central nervous system depressant agents) can lead to increased sedative (and sometimes depressive) effects.
Medications affecting sinus node function or atrio-ventricular nodal function (e.g. beta blockers, calcium channel blockers, digitalis)	Concomitant administration of Clonidine and medications affecting sinus node function or atrio-ventricular nodal function can result in bradycardia or atrio-ventricular block.
Tricyclic antidepressant medications and Prazosin	The hypotensive effects of Clonidine may be decreased.

Special Populations

The main recommendations for the use of Clonidine in patients with hepatic and renal impairment are shown in Table 5.8.

Table 5.8 Main recommendations for the use of Clonidine in patients with hepatic and renal impairment

Hepatic impairment	Use with caution (no known effects).
Renal impairment	Use with caution and consider reducing the dose of Clonidine, as its clearance is reduced in patients with severe renal insufficiency.

The main recommendations for the use of Clonidine during pregnancy and breastfeeding are shown in Table 5.9.

Table 5.9 Main recommendations for the use of Clonidine during pregnancy and breastfeeding

Pregnancy	Animal reproduction studies have shown adverse effects on the foetus and there are no controlled studies in humans, but potential benefits may warrant use of the medication in pregnant women despite potential risks, including lower foetal heart rate (former FDA Pregnancy Category C).
Breastfeeding	Evidence of excretion of Clonidine into breast milk: no adverse effects have been reported in nursing infants. If irritability or sedation develop in nursing infant, consider gradually discontinuing Clonidine or bottle feeding.

Behavioural Neurology

Initially developed as an anti-hypertensive medication, Clonidine is widely used for the treatment of neurodevelopmental conditions, such as attention-deficit and hyperactivity disorder (non-stimulant pharmacotherapy). With regard to tic control, Clonidine has been found to be less effective but better tolerated than anti-dopaminergic medications. The most commonly reported adverse effects are relatively mild and include dose-dependent sedation and hypotension. In consideration of its favourable tolerability profile, Clonidine has been proposed as a good initial choice for patients with disabling tics, especially in patients with co-morbid behavioural problems. It has also been shown that Clonidine may be particularly helpful in targeting irritability and aggressive/impulsive behaviours (including anger outbursts) associated with both Tourette syndrome and attention-deficit and hyperactivity disorder.

Guidelines

The main recommendations for the use of Clonidine according to the clinical guidelines on the treatment of tics are shown in Table 5.10.

Table 5.10 Main recommendations for the use of Clonidine according to published guidelines on the treatment of tics

Country (year)	Recommendation about Clonidine	Population
EU (+UK) (2011)	Evidence Level A (with attention-deficit and hyperactivity disorder as additional indication); included as second medication in survey of preferred choices	Children + adults
EU (+UK) (2012)[a]	Included as second medication in top three recommendations (children)	Children + adults
Canada (2012)	Strong recommendation, moderate-quality evidence	Children + adults
US (2013)	Listed with comments on adverse effects (sedation) and appropriateness of use in patients with initial insomnia (FDA-approved indication for attention-deficit and hyperactivity disorder)	Children
UK (2016)	Moderate certainty in the effect estimate (children) (downgraded because of suboptimal sample size)	Children
Japan (2019)[a]	[not included as first/second choice]	Children + adults
US (2019)	Moderate certainty in the effect estimate (children + adults) (based on one Class I study + two Class II studies)	Children + adults

[a] Expert survey and consensus.

Overall Rating

A summary of the efficacy and tolerability profiles of Clonidine in patients with Tourette syndrome is presented in Table 5.11.

Table 5.11 Summary of efficacy and tolerability profiles of Clonidine in patients with Tourette syndrome

Efficacy for tics	☺☺
Efficacy for behavioural problems	☺☺
Tolerability	☺☺☺

☺☺☺ = very good
☺☺ = good
☺ = acceptable

Guanfacine

Pharmacological Properties

The main pharmacodynamic and pharmacokinetic properties of Guanfacine (Figure 5.2) are summarized in Table 5.12.

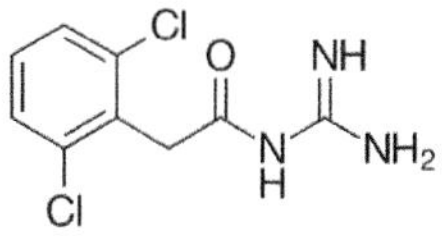

Figure 5.2 Guanfacine.

Table 5.12 Main pharmacodynamic and pharmacokinetic properties of Guanfacine

Mechanism(s) of action

Agonism of alpha-2A adrenergic receptors

Pharmacokinetics

Peak effect in approximately 3 hours (immediate release) or 6 hours (extended release)

Elimination half-life of approximately 17 hours

Half metabolized by liver (CYP450 3A4) into inactive metabolites and half eliminated unchanged in urine

Preparations

The relevant medicinal forms of Guanfacine are shown in Table 5.13.

Table 5.13 Relevant medicinal forms of Guanfacine

Tablets
Guanfacine 1 mg (immediate release)
Guanfacine 2 mg (immediate release)
Guanfacine 3 mg (immediate release)
Guanfacine 4 mg (immediate release)
Guanfacine 1 mg (extended release)
Guanfacine 2 mg (extended release)
Guanfacine 3 mg (extended release)
Guanfacine 4 mg (extended release)

Dose Titration

Dose is 1 mg daily for 14 days, then increased by 1 mg every 14 days; usual maintenance 1–2 mg once daily (immediate release) or 1–7 mg once daily (extended release) (maximum dose 7 mg daily).

Other Indications

The main clinical indications of Guanfacine in addition to tics are listed in Table 5.14.

Table 5.14 Main clinical indications of Guanfacine in addition to tics

Central nervous system conditions
Attention-deficit and hyperactivity disorder[a]
Irritability and aggressiveness
Anxiety
Alcohol and opiate withdrawal syndrome
Other conditions
Hypertension[a]

[a] FDA approved.

Cautions

Caution is warranted when using Guanfacine in patients with the conditions listed in Table 5.15.

Table 5.15 Cautions about the use of Guanfacine

Central nervous system conditions
–

Other conditions
Bradycardia, heart block
Cerebrovascular disease
Chronic renal or hepatic failure
History of cardiovascular disease
History of QT interval prolongation
Hypokalaemia
Recent myocardial infarction
Severe coronary insufficiency

Adverse Effects

The overall tolerability of Guanfacine in terms of sedation and weight gain is shown in Table 5.16, whereas the frequency of individual adverse effects is presented in Table 5.17.

Table 5.16 Overall tolerability of Guanfacine in terms of sedation and weight gain

Sedation	☹☹
Weight gain	–

☹☹☹ = significant problem
☹☹ = frequently reported
☹ = occasionally reported

Table 5.17 Frequency of adverse effects associated with Guanfacine

Very common (>1 in 10 patients on Guanfacine)	
CENTRAL NERVOUS SYSTEM:	OTHER SYSTEMS:
– Fatigue	– Abdominal pain
– Headache	
– Somnolence	

Common (>1 in 100 patients on Guanfacine)	
CENTRAL NERVOUS SYSTEM:	OTHER SYSTEMS:
– Affect lability	– Abdominal discomfort
– Anxiety	– Bradycardia
– Depression	– Constipation
– Dizziness	– Decreased appetite

Table 5.17 (cont.)

Common (>1 in 100 patients on Guanfacine)

– Insomnia	– Diarrhoea
– Irritability	– Dry mouth
– Lethargy	– Enuresis
– Nightmares	– Hypotension
– Sedation	– Nausea and vomiting
	– Skin rash
	– Weight gain

Uncommon (>1 in 1000 patients on Guanfacine)

CENTRAL NERVOUS SYSTEM:	OTHER SYSTEMS:
– Agitation	– Asthma
– Asthenia	– Atrio-ventricular block
– Hallucinations	– Chest pain
– Postural dizziness	– Dyspepsia
– Seizures	– Liver enzyme abnormalities
	– Pallor
	– Pollakiuria
	– Pruritus
	– Sinus arrhythmia
	– Syncope
	– Tachycardia

Rare (>1 in 10 000 patients on Guanfacine)

CENTRAL NERVOUS SYSTEM:	OTHER SYSTEMS:
– Hypersomnia	– Hypertension
	– Malaise

Very rare (<1 in 10 000 patients on Guanfacine)

CENTRAL NERVOUS SYSTEM:	OTHER SYSTEMS:
– Hypertensive encephalopathy	–

Interactions

The most relevant clinical interactions between Guanfacine and alcohol/other medications are shown in Table 5.18.

Table 5.18 Most relevant clinical interactions between Guanfacine and alcohol/other medications

Agent	Effect
Alcohol and central nervous system depressant agents	Concomitant administration of Guanfacine and alcohol (or other central nervous system depressant agents) can lead to increased sedative (and sometimes depressive) effects.
CYP450 3A inducers (e.g. Carbamazepine, glucocorticoids, Phenobarbital, Phenytoin, Rifampin, St John's wort)	Concomitant administration of Guanfacine and CYP450 3A inducers may result in lowered Guanfacine levels because of its increased clearance.

Table 5.18 (cont.)

Agent	Effect
CYP450 3A inhibitors (e.g. azole anti-fungals, Fluoxetine, Fluvoxamine, Ketoconazole, macrolides, Nefazodone, protease inhibitors)	Concomitant administration of Guanfacine and CYP450 3A inhibitors may result in raised Guanfacine levels because of tis decreased clearance.
High-fat meals	Exposure to Guanfacine (extended release) may be increased.
Valproate	Guanfacine may increase its plasma concentration.

Special Populations

The main recommendations for the use of Guanfacine in patients with hepatic and renal impairment are shown in Table 5.19.

Table 5.19 Main recommendations for the use of Guanfacine in patients with hepatic and renal impairment

Hepatic impairment	Use with caution and consider dose reduction in patients with significant impairment of hepatic function.
Renal impairment	Consider dose reduction in patients with severe impairment and end-stage renal disease.

The main recommendations for the use of Guanfacine during pregnancy and breast-feeding are shown in Table 5.20.

Table 5.20 Main recommendations for the use of Guanfacine during pregnancy and breastfeeding

Pregnancy	Not known to be harmful and not associated with increased risk of major congenital malformations; however, use of Guanfacine in women of childbearing potential requires weighing potential benefits to the mother against potential risks to the foetus (former FDA Pregnancy Category B).
Breastfeeding	Evidence of excretion of Guanfacine into breast milk (animal studies – unknown if Guanfacine is secreted in human breast milk): recommended to avoid.

Behavioural Neurology

Like Clonidine, Guanfacine is an alpha-2 adrenergic medication that is widely used for the treatment of neurodevelopmental conditions such as attention-deficit and hyperactivity disorder (non-stimulant pharmacotherapy). With regard to tic control, Guanfacine has been found to be less effective but better tolerated than anti-dopaminergic medications. Overall, the use of Guanfacine for the treatment of tics is not as well studied as the use of Clonidine. The most commonly reported adverse effects are relatively mild and include dose-dependent somnolence, hypotension and gastrointestinal symptoms. Guanfacine is relatively more selective for alpha2A receptors than Clonidine, potentially suggesting a more selective therapeutic action and an improved tolerability profile. Guanfacine may be particularly helpful in targeting irritability and aggressive/impulsive behaviours (including anger outbursts) associated with both Tourette syndrome and attention-deficit and hyperactivity disorder.

Guidelines

The main recommendations for the use of Guanfacine according to the clinical guidelines on the treatment of tics are shown in Table 5.21.

Table 5.21 Main recommendations for the use of Guanfacine according to published guidelines on the treatment of tics

Country (year)	Recommendation about Guanfacine	Population
EU (+UK) (2011)	Evidence Level A (with attention-deficit and hyperactivity disorder as additional indication); not included in top three recommendations in survey of preferred choices	Children + adults
EU (+UK) (2012)[a]	Not included in top three recommendations	Children + adults
Canada (2012)	Strong recommendation, moderate-quality evidence (children)	Children + adults
US (2013)	Listed with comments on support for use in patients with co-morbid attention-deficit and hyperactivity disorder (FDA-approved indication for attention-deficit and hyperactivity disorder)	Children
UK (2016)	Moderate certainty in the effect estimate (children) (downgraded because of suboptimal sample size)	Children
Japan (2019)[a]	Not included as first/second choice	Children + adults
US (2019)	Low certainty in the effect estimate (children) (based on one Class I study + two Class II studies – confidence in evidence downgraded due to imprecision)	Children + adults

[a] Expert survey and consensus.

Overall Rating

A summary of the efficacy and tolerability profiles of Guanfacine in patients with Tourette syndrome is presented in Table 5.22.

Table 5.22 Summary of efficacy and tolerability profiles of Guanfacine in patients with Tourette syndrome

Efficacy for tics	☺☺
Efficacy for behavioural problems	☺☺
Tolerability	☺☺☺

☺☺☺ = very good
☺☺ = good
☺ = acceptable

Other Tic-Suppressing Medications

Metoclopramide

Pharmacological Properties

The main pharmacodynamic and pharmacokinetic properties of Metoclopramide (Figure 6.1) are summarized in Table 6.1.

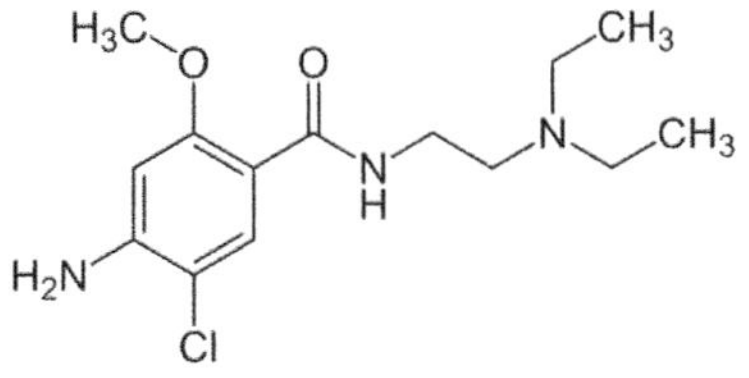

Figure 6.1 Metoclopramide.

Table 6.1 Main pharmacodynamic and pharmacokinetic properties of Metoclopramide

Mechanism(s) of action

Antagonism of dopamine D2 receptors

Antagonism of 5-HT3 serotonin receptors (at higher doses)

Agonism of 5-HT4 serotonin receptors

Pharmacokinetics

Peak effect in approximately 1–2 hours

Elimination half-life of approximately 6 hours

Mostly (85%) eliminated in urine

Preparations

The relevant medicinal forms of Metoclopramide are shown in Table 6.2.

Table 6.2 Relevant medicinal forms of Metoclopramide

Tablets

Metoclopramide 10 mg

Oral solution

Metoclopramide 1 mg/1 ml

Dose Titration

Dose is 10 mg daily for 14 days, then increased by 10 mg every 14 days; usual maintenance 30 mg daily in three divided doses (maximum dose 60 mg daily).

Other Indications

The main clinical indications of Metoclopramide in addition to tics are listed in Table 6.3.

Table 6.3 Main clinical indications of Metoclopramide in addition to tics

Central nervous system conditions

–

Other conditions

Diabetic gastroparesis[a]

Gastroesophageal reflux (short-term symptomatic treatment)[a]

Nausea, including that associated with palliative care and migraine (acute treatment)

[a] FDA approved.

Cautions

Caution is warranted when using Metoclopramide in patients with the conditions listed in Table 6.4.

Table 6.4 Cautions about the use of Metoclopramide

Central nervous system conditions

Parkinson disease

Other conditions

Gastrointestinal obstruction, haemorrhage or perforation[a]

Phaeochromocytoma[a]

Asthma, atopic allergy, bradycardia, cardiac conduction abnormalities, electrolyte imbalances

[a] Contraindication.

Adverse Effects

The overall tolerability of Metoclopramide in terms of sedation and weight gain is shown in Table 6.5, whereas the frequency of individual adverse effects is presented in Table 6.6.

Table 6.5 Overall tolerability of Metoclopramide in terms of sedation and weight gain

Sedation	☹
Weight gain	–

☹☹☹ = significant problem
☹☹ = frequently reported
☹ = occasionally reported

Table 6.6 Frequency of adverse effects associated with Metoclopramide

Very common (>1 in 10 patients on Metoclopramide)	
CENTRAL NERVOUS SYSTEM:	OTHER SYSTEMS:
– Sedation	

Common (>1 in 100 patients on Metoclopramide)	
CENTRAL NERVOUS SYSTEM:	OTHER SYSTEMS:
– Akathisia	– Diarrhoea
– Asthenia	– Hypotension
– Depression	– Menstrual disorder
– Extrapyramidal symptoms	

Uncommon (>1 in 1000 patients on Metoclopramide)	
CENTRAL NERVOUS SYSTEM:	OTHER SYSTEMS:
– Central nervous system depression	– Amenorrhoea
– Dyskinesias	– Arrhythmias
– Dystonia[a]	– Bradycardia
– Hallucinations	– Hyperprolactinaemia

Rare (>1 in 10 000 patients on Metoclopramide)	
CENTRAL NERVOUS SYSTEM:	OTHER SYSTEMS:
– Confusion	– Galactorrhoea
– Neuroleptic malignant syndrome	– Hepatotoxicity
– Seizures	– Skin reaction

Very rare (<1 in 10 000 patients on Metoclopramide)	
CENTRAL NERVOUS SYSTEM:	OTHER SYSTEMS:
–	–

[a] Plus unquantified risk of acute dystonic reactions (facial and skeletal muscle spasms and oculogyric crisis), especially in young female patients.

Interactions

The most relevant clinical interactions between Metoclopramide and alcohol/other medications are shown in Table 6.7.

Table 6.7 Most relevant clinical interactions between Metoclopramide and alcohol/other medications

Agent	Effect
Alcohol	Metoclopramide may increase its absorption and enhance its effects.
Cimetidine	Metoclopramide may decrease its effects because of decreased absorption (due to faster transit time).
Cyclosporine	Metoclopramide may increase its absorption and enhance its effects.
Digoxin	Metoclopramide may decrease its effects because of decreased absorption (due to faster transit time).
Levodopa	Metoclopramide increases its bioavailability due to increased absorption.
MAOIs	Metoclopramide releases catecholamines and may increase their effects.
Succinylcholine	Metoclopramide increases its neuromuscular blocking effects.

Special Populations

The main recommendations for the use of Metoclopramide in patients with hepatic and renal impairment are shown in Table 6.8.

Table 6.8 Main recommendations for the use of Metoclopramide in patients with hepatic and renal impairment

Hepatic impairment	Use with caution and reduce dose.
Renal impairment	Avoid or use small dose in severe impairment (decreased clearance and increased risk of extrapyramidal symptoms).

The main recommendations for the use of Metoclopramide during pregnancy and breastfeeding are shown in Table 6.9.

Table 6.9 Main recommendations for the use of Metoclopramide during pregnancy and breastfeeding

Pregnancy	Not known to be harmful and not associated with increased risk of major congenital malformations (former FDA Pregnancy Category B).
Breastfeeding	A small amount is present in breast milk: avoid or monitor infant for sedation.

Behavioural Neurology

In 2013 the benefits and risks of Metoclopramide were reviewed by the European Medicine Agency's Committee on Medicinal Products for Human Use, which concluded that the risk of neurological effects such as extrapyramidal symptoms and tardive dyskinesias outweigh the benefits in long-term or high-dose treatment. To help minimize the risk of potentially serious neurological adverse effects, specific restrictions were made to the use of Metoclopramide for the management of nausea and vomiting for short-term use (up to 5 days, maximum dose 0.5 mg/kg daily). Metoclopramide for the treatment of tics seems to be associated with overall better tolerability (less sedation or weight gain) than other anti-dopaminergic agents; however, the evidence for its effectiveness is considerably less strong.

Guidelines

The main recommendations for the use of Metoclopramide according to the clinical guidelines on the treatment of tics are shown in Table 6.10.

Table 6.10 Main recommendations for the use of Metoclopramide according to published guidelines on the treatment of tics

Country (year)	Recommendation about Metoclopramide	Population
EU (+UK) (2011)	Listed among alternative options; not included in top three recommendations in survey of preferred choices	Children + adults
EU (+UK) (2012)[a]	Not included in top three recommendations	Children + adults
Canada (2012)	Weak recommendation, low-quality evidence (children)	Children + adults
US (2013)	Not listed	Children
UK (2016)	Moderate certainty in the effect estimate (children) (downgraded because of suboptimal sample size and high risk of bias)	Children
Japan (2019)[a]	Not included as first/second choice	Children + adults
US (2019)	Low certainty in the effect estimate (children) (based on one Class II study)	Children + adults

[a] Expert survey and consensus.

Overall Rating

A summary of the efficacy and tolerability profiles of Metoclopramide in patients with Tourette syndrome is presented in Table 6.11.

Table 6.11 Summary of efficacy and tolerability profiles of Metoclopramide in patients with Tourette syndrome

Efficacy for tics	☺
Efficacy for behavioural problems	-
Tolerability	☺☺

☺☺☺ = very good
☺☺ = good
☺ = acceptable

Sulpiride

Pharmacological Properties

The main pharmacodynamic and pharmacokinetic properties of Sulpiride (Figure 6.2) are summarized in Table 6.12.

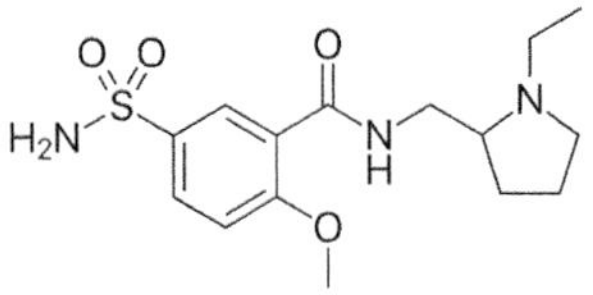

Figure 6.2 Sulpiride.

Table 6.12 Main pharmacodynamic and pharmacokinetic properties of Sulpiride

Mechanism(s) of action

Antagonism of D2, D3, D4 dopamine receptors

Pharmacokinetics

Peak effect in approximately 3–6 hours

Elimination half-life of approximately 7 hours

Eliminated in both urine and faeces largely (95%) unchanged

Preparations

The relevant medicinal forms of Sulpiride are shown in Table 6.13.

Dose Titration

Dose is 200 mg daily for 14 days, then increased by 200 mg every 14 days; usual maintenance 400–800 mg daily in two divided doses (maximum dose 2400 mg daily).

Table 6.13 Relevant medicinal forms of Sulpiride

Tablets

Sulpiride 200 mg

Sulpiride 400 mg

Oral solution

Sulpiride 40 mg/1 ml

Other Indications

The main clinical indications of Sulpiride in addition to tics are listed in Table 6.14.

Table 6.14 Main clinical indications of Sulpiride in addition to tics

Central nervous system conditions

Schizophrenia

Depression

Anxiety

Other conditions

–

Cautions

Caution is warranted when using Sulpiride in patients with the conditions listed in Table 6.15.

Table 6.15 Cautions about the use of Sulpiride

Central nervous system conditions

Central nervous system depression[a]

Prolactin-dependent tumours[a]

Aggression, agitation, mania

Alcohol withdrawal, seizures

Parkinson disease, Lewy body dementia

Other conditions

Phaeochromocytoma[a]

Cardiovascular disease, glaucoma, hypertension, hyperthyroidism, pulmonary disease, urinary retention

[a] Contraindication.

Adverse Effects

The overall tolerability of Sulpiride in terms of sedation and weight gain is shown in Table 6.16, whereas the frequency of individual adverse effects is presented in Table 6.17.

Table 6.16 Overall tolerability of Sulpiride in terms of sedation and weight gain

Sedation	☹☹
Weight gain	☹☹

☹☹☹ = significant problem
☹☹ = frequently reported
☹ = occasionally reported

Table 6.17 Frequency of adverse effects associated with Sulpiride

Very common (>1 in 10 patients on Sulpiride)	
CENTRAL NERVOUS SYSTEM:	OTHER SYSTEMS:
–	–

Common (>1 in 100 patients on Sulpiride)	
CENTRAL NERVOUS SYSTEM:	OTHER SYSTEMS:
– Akathisia	– Breast pain
– Extrapyramidal symptoms	– Constipation
– Insomnia	– Galactorrhoea
– Sedation	– Hyperprolactinaemia
– Tremor	– Liver enzyme abnormalities
	– Skin rash
	– Weight gain

Uncommon (>1 in 1000 patients on Sulpiride)	
CENTRAL NERVOUS SYSTEM:	OTHER SYSTEMS:
– Dizziness	– Amenorrhoea
– Dyskinesia	– Dry mouth
– Dystonia	– Erectile dysfunction
– Hypertonia	– Gynaecomastia
	– Hypersalivation
	– Leukopenia
	– Muscle stiffness
	– Nausea and vomiting
	– Orthostatic hypotension
	– Sexual dysfunction

Rare (>1 in 10 000 patients on Sulpiride)	
CENTRAL NERVOUS SYSTEM:	OTHER SYSTEMS:
– Neuroleptic malignant syndrome	– Ventricular tachycardia/ arrhythmia/fibrillation

Table 6.17 (cont.)

Rare (>1 in 10 000 patients on Sulpiride)
– Oculogyric crisis
– Seizures
– Tardive dyskinesias

Very rare (<1 in 10 000 patients on Sulpiride)	
CENTRAL NERVOUS SYSTEM:	OTHER SYSTEMS:
–	–

Interactions

The most relevant clinical interactions between Sulpiride and alcohol/other medications are shown in Table 6.18.

Table 6.18 Most relevant clinical interactions between Sulpiride and alcohol/other medications

Agent	Effect
Alcohol	Concomitant administration of Sulpiride and alcohol may increase the risk of central nervous system depression.
Antacids, Sucralfate	The absorption of Sulpiride may be reduced.
Anti-hypertensive medications	Sulpiride may increase their effects.
Levodopa and dopamine-agonists	Sulpiride may decrease their effects.

Special Populations

The main recommendations for the use of Sulpiride in patients with hepatic and renal impairment are shown in Table 6.19.

Table 6.19 Main recommendations for the use of Sulpiride in patients with hepatic and renal impairment

Hepatic impairment	Use with caution, as Sulpiride may precipitate coma.
Renal impairment	Use with caution as Sulpiride is eliminated by the renal route (start with small doses in patients with severe renal impairment because of increased cerebral sensitivity).

The main recommendations for the use of Sulpiride during pregnancy and breastfeeding are shown in Table 6.20.

Table 6.20 Main recommendations for the use of Sulpiride during pregnancy and breastfeeding

Pregnancy	Not known to be harmful and not associated with increased risk of major congenital malformations (former FDA Pregnancy Category B).
Breastfeeding	A small amount is present in breast milk: avoid or monitor infant for sedation.

Behavioural Neurology

Based on its pharmacological properties, Sulpiride is sometimes classed as a second-generation anti-dopaminergic medication. Sulpiride is poorly absorbed from the gastrointestinal tract and penetrates the blood-brain barrier with difficulty, leading to highly variable clinical responses. From the behavioural perspective, lower doses are more likely to be activating, whereas higher doses are more likely to be sedating. In addition to its established use for negative (lower doses) and positive (higher doses) psychotic symptoms, preliminary data on Sulpiride suggest some efficacy in anxiety and affective disorders (lower doses). There is evidence of potential usefulness for patients with Tourette syndrome; however, the use of Sulpiride for the treatment of tics is limited by its tolerability profile (especially dose-dependent sedation, metabolic dysfunction, and weight gain) and is not licensed in some countries (e.g. US).

Guidelines

The main recommendations for the use of Sulpiride according to the clinical guidelines on the treatment of tics are shown in Table 6.21.

Table 6.21 Main recommendations for the use of Sulpiride according to published guidelines on the treatment of tics

Country (year)	Recommendation about Sulpiride	Population
EU (+UK) (2011)	Evidence Level B (with obsessive-compulsive behaviour as additional indication); included as fifth medication in survey of preferred choices	Children + adults
EU (+UK) (2012)[a]	Included as third medication in top three recommendations (adults)	Children + adults
Canada (2012)	Not listed	Children + adults
US (2013)	Listed with comments on larger open-label paediatric study ($n = 189$) despite lack of approval in US	Children
UK (2016)	Not listed	Children
Japan (2019)[a]	Not included as first/second choice	Children + adults
US (2019)	Not listed	Children + adults

[a] Expert survey and consensus.

Overall Rating

A summary of the efficacy and tolerability profiles of Sulpiride in patients with Tourette syndrome is presented in Table 6.22.

Table 6.22 Summary of efficacy and tolerability profiles of Sulpiride in patients with Tourette syndrome

Efficacy for tics	☺☺
Efficacy for behavioural problems	☺☺
Tolerability	☺☺

☺☺☺ = very good
☺☺ = good
☺ = acceptable

Tetrabenazine

Pharmacological Properties

The main pharmacodynamic and pharmacokinetic properties of Tetrabenazine (Figure 6.3) are summarized in Table 6.23.

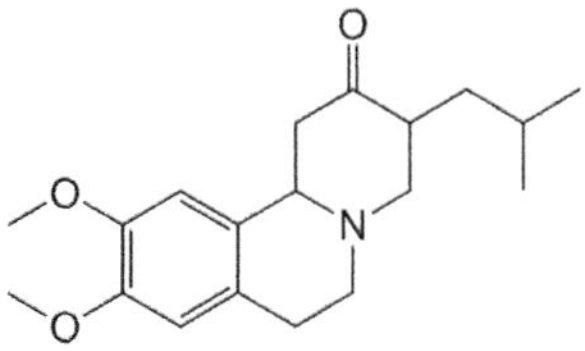

Figure 6.3 Tetrabenazine.

Table 6.23 Main pharmacodynamic and pharmacokinetic properties of Tetrabenazine

Mechanism(s) of action

Presynaptic depletion of monoamines (dopamine, as well as noradrenaline, serotonin and histadine) via reversible inhibition of vescicular monoamine transporter type 2 (VMAT2)

Antagonism of D2 dopamine receptors (weak effect)

Pharmacokinetics

Peak effect in approximately 2 hours

Elimination half-life of approximately 10 hours

Eliminated in both urine (75%) and faeces

Preparations

The relevant medicinal forms of Tetrabenazine are shown in Table 6.24.

Table 6.24 Relevant medicinal forms of Tetrabenazine

Tablets

Tetrabenazine 12.5 mg

Tetrabenazine 25 mg

Dose Titration

Dose is 12.5–25 mg daily for 14 days, then increased by 12.5–25 mg every 14 days; usual maintenance 37.5–75 mg daily in two to three divided doses (maximum dose 200 mg daily).

Other Indications

The main clinical indications of Tetrabenazine in addition to tics are listed in Table 6.25.

Table 6.25 Main clinical indications of Tetrabenazine in addition to tics

Central nervous system conditions

Chorea in Huntington disease[a]

Tardive dyskinesias

Dystonia

Hemiballism

Myoclonus

Psychosis

Other conditions

Hypertension

[a] FDA approved.

Cautions

Caution is warranted when using Tetrabenazine in patients with the conditions listed in Table 6.26.

Table 6.26 Cautions about the use of Tetrabenazine

Central nervous system conditions

Concomitant administration of MAOIs or Reserpine[a]

Depression[a]

Hepatic disorders[a]

Parkinson disease[a], parkinsonism[a]

Prolactin-dependent tumours[a]

Other conditions

Phaeochromocytoma[a]

Susceptibility to QT interval prolongation

[a] Contraindication.

Adverse Effects

The overall tolerability of Tetrabenazine in terms of sedation and weight gain is shown in Table 6.27, whereas the frequency of individual adverse effects is presented in Table 6.28.

Table 6.27 Overall tolerability of Tetrabenazine in terms of sedation and weight gain

Sedation	☹☹
Weight gain	☹☹

☹☹☹ = significant problem
☹☹ = frequently reported
☹ = occasionally reported

Table 6.28 Frequency of adverse effects associated with Tetrabenazine

Very common (>1 in 10 patients on Tetrabenazine)	
CENTRAL NERVOUS SYSTEM:	OTHER SYSTEMS:
– Depression	–
– Extrapyramidal symptoms	
– Sedation	

Common (>1 in 100 patients on Tetrabenazine)	
CENTRAL NERVOUS SYSTEM:	OTHER SYSTEMS:
– Anxiety	– Constipation
– Confusion	– Diarrhoea
– Dizziness	– Dysphagia
– Fatigue	– Hypotension
– Insomnia	– Nausea and vomiting
	– Weight gain

Uncommon (>1 in 1000 patients on Tetrabenazine)	
CENTRAL NERVOUS SYSTEM:	OTHER SYSTEMS:
– Central nervous system depression	– Autonomic dysfunction
	– Hyperthermia
	– Muscle stiffness

Rare (>1 in 10 000 patients on Tetrabenazine)	
CENTRAL NERVOUS SYSTEM:	OTHER SYSTEMS:
– Neuroleptic malignant syndrome	

Very rare (<1 in 10 000 patients on Tetrabenazine)	
CENTRAL NERVOUS SYSTEM:	OTHER SYSTEMS:
–	– Skeletal muscle damage

Interactions

The most relevant clinical interactions between Tetrabenazine and alcohol/other medications are shown in Table 6.29.

Table 6.29 Most relevant clinical interactions between Tetrabenazine and alcohol/other medications

Agent	Effect
Alcohol	Concomitant administration of Tetrabenazine and alcohol may increase the risk of central nervous system depression and sedation.
CYP450 2D6 stronger inhibitors (e.g. Fluoxetine, Paroxetine, Quinidine)	Concomitant administration of Tetrabenazine and CYP450 2D6 stronger inhibitors may result in raised Tetrabenazine levels (doubling), requiring reduction in dose.
CYP450 2D6 weaker inhibitors (e.g. Amiodarone, Duloxetine, Sertraline)	Concomitant administration of Tetrabenazine and CYP450 2D6 weaker inhibitors may result in raised Tetrabenazine levels.
CYP450 2D6 inducers (e.g. Dexamethasone, Rifampin)	Concomitant administration of Tetrabenazine and CYP450 2D6 inducers may result in reduced Tetrabenazine levels.

Special Populations

The main recommendations for the use of Tetrabenazine in patients with hepatic and renal impairment are shown in Table 6.30.

Table 6.30 Main recommendations for the use of Tetrabenazine in patients with hepatic and renal impairment

Hepatic impairment	Use with caution in mild to moderate impairment (use half initial dose and slower dose titration); avoid in severe impairment, as the concentration and half-life of Tetrabenazine and its metabolites can be considerably increased.
Renal impairment	Use with caution, as patients with renal insufficiency may adjust poorly to lowered blood pressure resulting from Tetrabenazine use.

The main recommendations for the use of Tetrabenazine during pregnancy and breast-feeding are shown in Table 6.31.

Table 6.31 Main recommendations for the use of Tetrabenazine during pregnancy and breastfeeding

Pregnancy	Animal reproduction studies have shown adverse effects on the foetus and there are no controlled studies in humans, but potential benefits may warrant use of the medication in pregnant women despite potential risks (former FDA Pregnancy Category C).
Breastfeeding	Unknown if it is secreted in breast milk: avoid unless clearly needed.

Behavioural Neurology

Tetrabenazine is a presynaptic depletor of monoamines with a better tolerability profile than Reserpine (shorter half-life and fewer peripheral effects, such as gastrointestinal symptoms and hypotension). Extrapyramidal symptoms and weight gain are less common and QT interval prolongation is milder compared to most first-generation anti-dopaminergic medications. In addition to its established use in the treatment of hyperkinetic movement disorders, Tetrabenazine has been shown to have clinically significant behavioural effects. There is evidence that Tetrabenazine may be effective in the treatment of tics, although its use in patients with Tourette syndrome is limited by its adverse effects, including sedation and depression.

Guidelines

The main recommendations for the use of Tetrabenazine according to the clinical guidelines on the treatment of tics are shown in Table 6.32.

Table 6.32 Main recommendations for the use of Tetrabenazine according to published guidelines on the treatment of tics

Country (year)	Recommendation about Tetrabenazine	Population
EU (+UK) (2011)	Listed among alternative options; included as eighth medication in survey of preferred choices	Children + adults
EU (+UK) (2012)[a]	Not included in top three recommendations	Children + adults
Canada (2012)	Weak recommendation, very low quality evidence	Children + adults
US (2013)	Listed with comments on adverse effects (sedation, weight gain, depression)	Children
UK (2016)	Not listed	Children
Japan (2019)[a]	Not included as first/second choice	Children + adults
US (2019)	Listed as increasingly used off-label, possibly associated with adverse effects (sedation, depression and extrapyramidal symptoms)	Children + adults

[a] Expert survey and consensus.

Overall Rating

A summary of the efficacy and tolerability profiles of Tetrabenazine in patients with Tourette syndrome is presented in Table 6.33.

Table 6.33 Summary of efficacy and tolerability profiles of Tetrabenazine in patients with Tourette syndrome

Efficacy for tics	☺
Efficacy for behavioural problems	☺
Tolerability	☺

☺☺☺ = very good
☺☺ = good
☺ = acceptable

Tiapride

Pharmacological Properties

The main pharmacodynamic and pharmacokinetic properties of Tiapride (Figure 6.4) are summarized in Table 6.34.

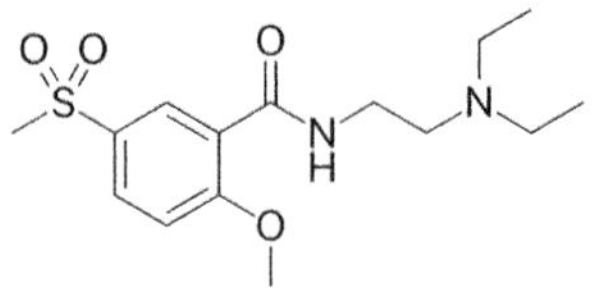

Figure 6.4 Tiapride.

Table 6.34 Main pharmacodynamic and pharmacokinetic properties of Tiapride

Mechanism(s) of action

Antagonism of D2, D3, D4 dopamine receptors

Pharmacokinetics

Peak effect in approximately 1 hour

Elimination half-life of approximately 3 hours

Mostly eliminated in urine

Preparations

The relevant medicinal forms of Tiapride are shown in Table 6.35.

Table 6.35 Relevant medicinal forms of Tiapride

Tablets

Tiapride 100 mg

Tiapride 200 mg

Dose Titration

Dose is 100 mg daily for 14 days, then increased by 100 mg every 14 days; usual maintenance 200–600 mg daily in two to three divided doses (maximum dose 1800 mg daily).

Other Indications

The main clinical indications of Tiapride in addition to tics are listed in Table 6.36.

Table 6.36 Main clinical indications of Tiapride in addition to tics

Central nervous system conditions

Tardive dyskinesias

Chorea

Anxiety

Alcohol withdrawal syndrome

Other conditions

—

Cautions

Caution is warranted when using Tiapride in patients with the conditions listed in Table 6.37.

Table 6.37 Cautions about the use of Tiapride

Central nervous system conditions

Central nervous system depression[a]

Prolactin-dependent tumours[a]

Alcohol withdrawal, seizures

Parkinson disease

Other conditions

Phaeochromocytoma[a]

[a] Contraindication.

Adverse Effects

The overall tolerability of Tiapride in terms of sedation and weight gain is shown in Table 6.38, whereas the frequency of individual adverse effects is presented in Table 6.39.

Table 6.38 Overall tolerability of Tiapride in terms of sedation and weight gain

Sedation	☹☹
Weight gain	☹☹

☹☹☹ = significant problem
☹☹ = frequently reported
☹ = occasionally reported

Table 6.39 Frequency of adverse effects associated with Tiapride

Very common (>1 in 10 patients on Tiapride)	
CENTRAL NERVOUS SYSTEM:	OTHER SYSTEMS:
–	–

Common (>1 in 100 patients on Tiapride)	
CENTRAL NERVOUS SYSTEM:	OTHER SYSTEMS:
– Agitation	– Hypersalivation
– Apathy	– Orthostatic hypotension
– Asthenia	
– Dizziness	
– Extrapyramidal symptoms	
– Headache	
– Hypokinesia	
– Insomnia	
– Sedation	
– Rigidity	
– Tremor	

Uncommon (>1 in 1000 patients on Tiapride)	
CENTRAL NERVOUS SYSTEM:	OTHER SYSTEMS:
– Akathisia	– Amenorrhoea/
– Acute dystonic reaction	dysmenorrhoea
– Oculogyric crisis	– Breast pain
	– Galactorrhoea
	– Gynaecomastia
	– Hyperprolactinaemia
	– Erectile dysfunction
	– Sexual dysfunction
	– Weight gain

Rare (>1 in 10 000 patients on Tiapride)	
CENTRAL NERVOUS SYSTEM:	OTHER SYSTEMS:
–	–

Very rare (<1 in 10 000 patients on Tiapride)	
CENTRAL NERVOUS SYSTEM:	OTHER SYSTEMS:
– Neuroleptic malignant syndrome	–
– Tardive dyskinesias	

Interactions

The most relevant clinical interactions between Tiapride and alcohol/other medications are shown in Table 6.40.

Table 6.40 Most relevant clinical interactions between Tiapride and alcohol/other medications

Agent	Effect
Alcohol	Concomitant administration of Tiapride and alcohol may increase the risk of central nervous system depression.
Anti-cholinergics (e.g. Biperiden)	The action of Tiapride may be attenuated.
Central nervous system depressant agents (e.g. anxiolytics, barbiturates, benzodiazepines, centrally acting anti-hypertensive medications such as Clonidine and Guanfacine, H1 anti-histaminergic medications)	Tiapride may increase their effects.
Levodopa and dopamine-agonists	Tiapride may decrease their effects.

Special Populations

The main recommendations for the use of Tiapride in patients with hepatic and renal impairment are shown in Table 6.41.

Table 6.41 Main recommendations for the use of Tiapride in patients with hepatic and renal impairment

Hepatic impairment	Use with caution.
Renal impairment	Use with caution, as Tiapride is eliminated by the renal route (start with small doses in patients with severe renal impairment because of increased cerebral sensitivity).

The main recommendations for the use of Tiapride during pregnancy and breastfeeding are shown in Table 6.42.

Table 6.42 Main recommendations for the use of Tiapride during pregnancy and breastfeeding

Pregnancy	Not known to be harmful and not associated with increased risk of major congenital malformations (former FDA Pregnancy Category B).
Breastfeeding	A small amount is present in breast milk: avoid or monitor infant for sedation.

Behavioural Neurology

Based on its pharmacological properties, Tiapride is sometimes classed as a second-generation anti-dopaminergic medication, like the other substituted benzamide Sulpiride. The main clinical indications of Tiapride include tardive dyskinesias, chorea, anxiety and alcohol withdrawal syndrome. There is evidence of potential usefulness for patients with Tourette syndrome; however, the use of Tiapride for the treatment of tics is limited by its tolerability profile (especially dose-dependent sedation, metabolic dysfunction and weight gain) and is not licensed in some countries (e.g. US).

Guidelines

The main recommendations for the use of Tiapride according to the clinical guidelines on the treatment of tics are shown in Table 6.43.

Table 6.43 Main recommendations for the use of Tiapride according to published guidelines on the treatment of tics

Country (year)	Recommendation about Tiapride	Population
EU (+UK) (2011)	Evidence Level B; included as sixth medication in survey of preferred choices	Children + adults
EU (+UK) (2012)[a]	Not listed	Children + adults
Canada (2012)	Not listed	Children + adults
US (2013)	Listed despite lack of approval in US	Children
UK (2016)	Not listed	Children
Japan (2019)[a]	Not included as first/second choice	Children + adults
US (2019)	Moderate certainty in the effect estimate (children) (based on one Class I study)	Children + adults

[a] Expert survey and consensus.

Overall Rating

A summary of the efficacy and tolerability profiles of Tiapride in patients with Tourette syndrome is presented in Table 6.44.

Table 6.44 Summary of efficacy and tolerability profiles of Tiapride in patients with Tourette syndrome

Efficacy for tics	☺☺
Efficacy for behavioural problems	☺☺
Tolerability	☺☺

☺☺☺ = very good
☺☺ = good
☺ = acceptable

Topiramate

Pharmacological Properties

The main pharmacodynamic and pharmacokinetic properties of Topiramate (Figure 6.5) are summarized in Table 6.45.

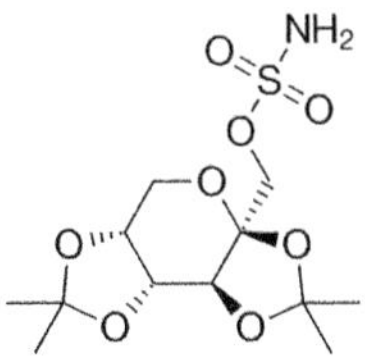

Figure 6.5 Topiramate.

Table 6.45 Main pharmacodynamic and pharmacokinetic properties of Topiramate

Mechanism(s) of action

Blockade of voltage-dependent sodium channels

Potentiation of GABA-A1 mediated neurotransmission

Antagonism of glutamate receptors (AMPA subtype)

Inhibition of carbonic anhydrase isoenzymes (II and IV)

Blockade of calcium channels

Inhibition of protein kinase activity

Pharmacokinetics

Peak effect in approximately 2 hours

Elimination half-life of approximately 21 hours

Mostly (70%–80%) eliminated in urine

Preparations

The relevant medicinal forms of Topiramate are shown in Table 6.46.

Table 6.46 Relevant medicinal forms of Topiramate

Tablets

Topiramate 25 mg

Topiramate 50 mg

Topiramate 100 mg

Topiramate 200 mg

Capsules

Topiramate 15 mg

Topiramate 25 mg

Topiramate 50 mg

Other Indications

The main clinical indications of Topiramate in addition to tics are listed in Table 6.47.

Table 6.47 Main clinical indications of Topiramate in addition to tics

Central nervous system conditions

Epilepsy[a]

Migraine prophylaxis[a]

Essential tremor

Bipolar affective disorder

Binge-eating disorder/bulimia

Other conditions

Obesity (in combination with Phentermine)[a]

Neuropathic pain

[a] FDA approved.

Dose Titration

Dose is 25 mg nocte for 14 days, then increased by 25–50 mg every 14 days; usual maintenance 100–200 mg daily in two divided doses (maximum dose 500 mg daily, although doses of 1000 mg daily have been used for refractory epilepsy)

Cautions

Caution is warranted when using Topiramate in patients with the conditions listed in Table 6.48.

Table 6.48 Cautions about the use of Topiramate

Central nervous system conditions

—

Other conditions

Acute porphyrias[a]

Risk factors for metabolic acidosis

Risk factors for nephrolithiasis (ensure adequate hydration)

[a] Contraindication.

Adverse Effects

The overall tolerability of Topiramate in terms of sedation and weight gain is shown in Table 6.49, whereas the frequency of individual adverse effects is presented in Table 6.50.

Table 6.49 Overall tolerability of Topiramate in terms of sedation and weight gain

Sedation	☹☹
Weight gain	–

☹☹☹ = significant problem
☹☹ = frequently reported
☹ = occasionally reported

Table 6.50 Frequency of adverse effects associated with Topiramate

Very common (>1 in 10 patients on Topiramate)	
CENTRAL NERVOUS SYSTEM:	OTHER SYSTEMS:
– Depression	– Diarrhoea
– Dizziness	– Nausea
– Fatigue	– Weight loss
– Paraesthesias	
– Sedation	

Common (>1 in 100 patients on Topiramate)	
CENTRAL NERVOUS SYSTEM:	OTHER SYSTEMS:
– Aggression	– Abdominal pain
– Agitation	– Alopecia
– Anxiety	– Anaemia
– Ataxia	– Arthralgia
– Cognitive impairment	– Constipation
– Confusion	– Dry mouth
– Impaired attention	– Dyspepsia
– Irritability	– Dyspnoea
– Mood changes	– Epistaxis
– Movement disorders	– Gastritis
– Nystagmus	– Malaise
– Seizures	– Muscle spasms/weakness/pain
– Sleep disturbance	
– Speech disorder	– Nephrolithiasis
– Taste disturbance	– Pruritus
– Tinnitus	– Skin rash
– Tremor	– Urinary disorders
– Visual disturbances	– Vomiting

Uncommon (>1 in 1000 patients on Topiramate)	
CENTRAL NERVOUS SYSTEM:	OTHER SYSTEMS:
– Altered sense of smell	– Abdominal distension
– Hearing loss	– Blepharospasm
– Mydriasis	– Blood disorders

Table 6.50 (cont.)

Uncommon (>1 in 1000 patients on Topiramate)	
– Panic attacks	– Bradycardia
– Photophobia	– Dry eye
– Psychosis	– Flatulence
– Suicidal ideation	– Flushing
– Thirst	– Gingival bleeding
	– Glossodynia
	– Haematuria
	– Halitosis
	– Hypersalivation
	– Hypokalaemia
	– Hypotension and postural hypotension
	– Increased lacrimation
	– Influenza-like symptoms
	– Leukopenia
	– Metabolic acidosis
	– Neutropenia
	– Palpitation
	– Pancreatitis
	– Peripheral neuropathy
	– Reduced sweating
	– Sexual dysfunction
	– Skin discoloration
	– Thrombocytopenia
	– Urinary calculus

Rare (>1 in 10 000 patients on Topiramate)	
CENTRAL NERVOUS SYSTEM:	OTHER SYSTEMS:
– Unilateral blindness	– Abnormal skin odour
	– Calcinosis
	– Hepatic failure and hepatitis
	– Periorbital oedema
	– Raynaud phenomenon
	– Severe skin reaction (Stevens–Johnson syndrome)

Very rare (<1 in 10 000 patients on Topiramate)	
CENTRAL NERVOUS SYSTEM:	OTHER SYSTEMS:
–	– Angle-closure glaucoma[a]

[a] Acute myopia with secondary angle-closure glaucoma, typically occurring within 1 month of starting Topiramate (choroidal effusions resulting in anterior displacement of the lens and iris have also been reported).

Interactions

The most relevant clinical interactions between Topiramate and alcohol/other medications are shown in Table 6.51.

Table 6.51 Most relevant clinical interactions between Topiramate and alcohol/other medications

Agent	Effect
Acetazolamide (and other carbonic anhydrase inhibitors)	Concomitant administration of Topiramate and carbonic anhydrase inhibitors increases the risk of metabolic acidosis and kidney stones.
Alcohol	Concomitant administration of Topiramate and alcohol (or other central nervous system depressant agents) has not been evaluated in clinical studies: their concomitant use is not recommended.
Amitriptyline, Phenytoin	Topiramate may increase their plasma concentration.
Carbamazepine, Phenytoin, Pioglitazone, Valproate	The plasma concentration of Topiramate may be decreased, as its clearance may be increased.
Digoxin Lithium, Valproate	Topiramate may decrease their plasma concentration.
Hydrochlorothiazide, Lamotrigine	The plasma concentration of Topiramate may be increased.
Oestrogens and progestins	Higher-dose Topiramate may decrease their plasma concentration.

Special Populations

The main recommendations for the use of Topiramate in patients with hepatic and renal impairment are shown in Table 6.52.

Table 6.52 Main recommendations for the use of Topiramate in patients with hepatic and renal impairment

Hepatic impairment	Use with caution in moderate to severe impairment, as Topiramate clearance may be reduced.
Renal impairment	Use with caution as the plasma and renal clearance of Topiramate may be decreased and patients may require a longer time to reach steady-state at each dose (half of the usual starting and maintenance dose is recommended).

The main recommendations for the use of Topiramate during pregnancy and breast-feeding are shown in Table 6.53.

Behavioural Neurology

In addition to its established use in epilepsy and migraine prophylaxis, preliminary data on Topiramate suggest some efficacy in obsessive-compulsive disorder, eating disorders (binge eating), behavioural and psychological symptoms of dementia, alcohol and cocaine

Table 6.53 Main recommendations for the use of Topiramate during pregnancy and breastfeeding

Pregnancy	Known to be associated with increased risk (3-fold for exposure to Topiramate monotherapy during the first trimester) of major congenital malformations (cleft lip/palate, hypospadias, and anomalies involving various body systems) and low birth weight. If potential benefits warrant use of Topiramate during the first trimester, careful prenatal monitoring should be performed (former FDA Pregnancy Category D).
Breastfeeding	Possibility of extensive excretion of Topiramate into breast milk based on limited observations: consider suspending breastfeeding or discontinuing/abstaining from Topiramate therapy.

dependence. There is also some evidence that this medication may be effective in the treatment of depression, either as monotherapy or as adjunctive treatment. The findings of initial reports suggesting that Topiramate can be effective in the treatment of bipolar affective disorder and post-traumatic stress disorders have not been confirmed by the results of randomized controlled trials. In 2012, Topiramate in combination with Phentermine received FDA approval for weight loss: this is a clinically significant effect in patients with tics and behavioural problems, as pharmacotherapy is often associated with metabolic dysfunction and weight gain. Topiramate for the treatment of tics could be a promising alternative option to both anti-dopaminergic and alpha-2 adrenergic agents, with an overall acceptable tolerability, although the evidence for its effectiveness is less strong.

Guidelines

The main recommendations for the use of Topiramate according to the clinical guidelines on the treatment of tics are shown in Table 6.54.

Table 6.54 Main recommendations for the use of Topiramate according to published guidelines on the treatment of tics

Country (year)	Recommendation about Topiramate	Population
EU (+UK) (2011)	Listed among alternative options; not included in top three recommendations in survey of preferred choices	Children + adults
EU (+UK) (2012)[a]	Not included in top three recommendations	Children + adults
Canada (2012)	Weak recommendation, low-quality evidence	Children + adults
US (2013)	Not listed	Children
UK (2016)	Low certainty in the effect estimate (children + adults)	Children

Table 6.54 (cont.)

Country (year)	Recommendation about Topiramate	Population
	(downgraded because of suboptimal sample size)	
Japan (2019)[a]	Not included as first/second choice	Children + adults
US (2019)	Low certainty in the effect estimate (children + adults) (based on one Class I study)	Children + adults

[a] Expert survey and consensus.

Overall Rating

A summary of the efficacy and tolerability profiles of Topiramate in patients with Tourette syndrome is presented in Table 6.55.

Table 6.55 Summary of efficacy and tolerability profiles of Topiramate in patients with Tourette syndrome

Efficacy for tics	☺☺
Efficacy for behavioural problems	☺
Tolerability	☺☺

☺☺☺ = very good
☺☺ = good
☺ = acceptable

Chapter

7 Guidelines Based on Systematic Literature Review and Meta-analysis

Over the last few decades, evidence-based medicine has established itself as a new paradigm for teaching and practising clinical medicine. Double-blind randomized controlled trials and high-quality observational studies have gradually replaced tradition, anecdote, and theoretical reasoning from basic sciences, as sources of evidence to complement clinical expertise in order to fulfil patients' needs. The development of disease-specific guidelines has arguably contributed to the process of making clinical practice more scientific and empirically grounded, resulting in safer, more consistent and more cost effective care. However the evidence-based paradigm has received criticism based on the argument that the emphasis on experimental evidence could devalue basic sciences and the tacit knowledge that accumulates with clinical experience. Moreover, it has been argued that the evidence-based movement arose primarily from a desire to standardize care, rather than individualizing it. Practising medicine according to the standards set out by guidelines could be seen as antithetical to practising according to clinical judgement: standardization can only identify best practices for an 'average' patient under 'average' conditions, whereas clinical judgement is by definition personal and seeks to decide what is best for a 'specific' patient at a 'specific' time. It has also been questioned whether findings from average results in clinical trials could inform decisions about real patients, who rarely fit the textbook description of disease and differ from those included in the research trials based on which guidelines are developed. In other words, evidence-based medicine could introduce an intrinsic bias due to its tendency to treat patients according to population norms rather than personal needs. The danger of a subtle shift from patient-centred to management-driven care provision is real, but can be controlled by a knowledgeable and compassionate practice of evidence-based medicine, capable of accommodating basic scientific principles, the subtleties of clinical judgement and the patient's individual idiosyncrasies.

Real evidence-based medicine should have the care of individual patients as its top priority. To support such an approach, evidence must be individualized for the patient: the question clinicians should ask themselves is 'what is the best course of action for this patient, in these circumstances, at this point in their condition?' The role of the clinician is the role of a skilful interpreter, in finding out what matters to the patient, and a wise adviser, in making judicious use of professional knowledge and introducing research evidence in a way that informs a dialogue about what would be best to do, how and why. Real evidence-based medicine should be characterized by expert judgement (rather than mechanical rule following) forming the basis of decision sharing with patients through meaningful conversations and of stronger clinician-patient relationships.

Clinicians who rely on evidence-based guidelines should not underestimate the human aspects of care. This is particularly relevant to Tourette syndrome, as current clinical guidelines are the result of evidence built on a limited number of randomized controlled trials relying on the use of placebo for the control group (Table 7.1).

Table 7.1 Guidelines on pharmacotherapy for patients with Tourette syndrome and other tic disorders published since 2010

Authors	Year	Journal	Country	Population	SLR/MA/EC
ESSTS	2011	*Eur J Child Adolesc Psychiatr*	EU (+UK)	Children + adults	SLR (four parts)
Rickards et al.	2012	*Eur J Paediatr Neurol*	EU (+UK)	Children + adults	EC
Pringsheim et al.	2012	*Can J Psychiatr*	Canada	Children + adults	SLR (two parts)
AACAP	2013	*J Am Acad Child Adolesc Psychiatr*	US	Children	SLR
Hollis et al.	2016	*Health Technol Assess*	UK	Children	SLR + MA
Hamamoto et al.	2019	*Brain Develop*	Japan	Children + adults	EC
AAN	2019	*Neurology*	US	Children + adults	SLR + MA

Abbreviations. AACAP, American Academy of Child and Adolescent Psychiatry; AAN, American Academy of Neurology; EC, expert survey and consensus; ESSTS, European Society for the Study of Tourette Syndrome; HTA, health technology assessment; MA, meta-analysis; SLR, systematic literature review.

Evidence-based guidelines are known to map poorly to patients presenting with complex co-morbidities. Statistically significant benefits observed in trials may be marginal in clinical practice. Crucially, in randomized controlled trials of medications for tics, placebos have often demonstrated substantial reduction in tic and tic-related impairments. It has been estimated that the placebo effect can account for 30 per cent of improvement in tic severity and 40 per cent of improvement in overall impairment in about 20 per cent of patients. Female patients have been shown to be more likely to have a significant placebo response. The role of placebos as robust tic suppressors suggests that there is therapeutic benefit for tics simply by intervening and highlights the importance of placebo-controlled trials to determine the efficacy of pharmacological agents for tics.

There is evidence that the placebo effect, a well-known and well-documented therapeutic phenomenon, is widely accepted and used by clinicians in patient care. Most patients favour the idea of placebo treatments and value honesty and transparency in this context, suggesting that clinicians should consider engaging in discussions about their therapeutic value. There is also evidence for positive parental support of appropriate placebo use in paediatric trials and in clinical settings for selected conditions, without the practice of deception and with the creation of guidelines for ethical and safe practice. This might be particularly relevant for younger patients with Tourette syndrome, as parents' perceptions have been shown to influence the placebo effect in their children.

Europe and UK (2011)

A set of four guidelines on the assessment and treatment of Tourette syndrome was published in the *European Journal of Child and Adolescent Psychiatry* by the members of the European Society for the Study of Tourette Syndrome (ESSTS), including the UK, in 2011. Specifically, the four documents covered the following topics: assessment (Part I), pharmacological treatment (Part II), behavioural and psychosocial interventions (Part III) and deep brain stimulation (Part IV). When asking which specific agents can be recommended for the treatment of tics in patients with Tourette syndrome, the authors of the ESSTS guidelines acknowledged the scarcity of studies directly comparing the efficacy and safety of different pharmacological agents, especially with regard to their longer-term effects. A systematic review of the existing literature confirmed that the best level of evidence arising from randomized, double-blind, placebo-controlled studies was still available for first-generation anti-dopaminergic agents, namely Haloperidol and Pimozide. There were some indications that Pimozide may be more effective and may have a somewhat more favourable adverse reaction profile than Haloperidol, with the exception of its potential cardiological adverse effects. However the authors acknowledged that in clinical practice across Europe, Haloperidol and Pimozide had been gradually replaced by second-generation anti-dopaminergic agents.

According to the ESSTS guidelines, the best evidence was available for Risperidone, the second-generation anti-dopaminergic agent with the larger number of reviewed studies. Although second-generation anti-dopaminergic medications had traditionally been associated with lower risk for adverse reactions, the authors pointed out that a few adverse reactions were similar to those associated with the use of first-generation anti-dopaminergic agents, including sedation, akathisia, weight gain, tardive dyskinesia and neuroleptic malignant syndrome. Second-generation anti-dopaminergic agents were generally associated with a lower incidence of extrapyramidal symptoms; however, it was noted that a rapid dose escalation increased the risk for such adverse events. Moreover, according to the authors the paucity of long-term studies in patients with Tourette syndrome suggested that the risks of metabolic syndromes and QTc prolongation could not be quantified. Although at the time of the publication of the ESSTS guidelines placebo-controlled studies with Aripiprazole were still missing, the authors referred to this medication as 'rather promising', in consideration of the lower risk of weight gain as adverse reaction and encouraging positive effects in patients who had not responded to previous treatments.

It was also noted that the substituted benzamides Sulpiride and Tiapride were commonly used as first-line agents to treat Tourette syndrome (particularly in children and adolescents) in the German-speaking world, but not in most other countries. Consequently, their clinical efficacy for tic control and their pharmacological properties had been under-investigated in comparison to other anti-dopaminergic compounds. Despite the small base of evidence, the authors referred to previous expert opinion that Sulpiride and Tiapride were highly recommendable to treat Tourette syndrome in view of their excellent balance of efficacy and tolerability proven over decades in clinical practice.

Finally, it was acknowledged that both tic severity and presence of co-morbid behavioural symptoms may affect the choice of medication. The authors stated that although the evidence in favour of the tic-suppressing effects of Clonidine might be less compelling compared to the anti-dopaminergic agents, this medication had the potential to actually improve attention-deficit and hyperactivity symptoms, as well as mild to moderate tics. It was noted that Clonidine was also useful to alleviate initial insomnia and reduce anxiety.

In consideration of the paucity of controlled clinical trials available for review, the authors highlighted that every general recommendation depends heavily on the experts' experiences and preferences. Therefore the authors sent a questionnaire to all clinicians with experience in the treatment of Tourette syndrome who were members of the ESSTS. Participants were asked what pharmacological agent they would consider as first, second, third and subsequent choice(s) in the treatment of tics for children and adolescents without co-morbid conditions. The authors sent out 60 questionnaires and rated each participant's first choice medication with 4 points, second choice with 3 points, third choice with 2 points and any additional medications with 1 point. The final scores, based on 22 responses, were as follows (top 10 medications): Risperidone 60, Clonidine 37, Aripiprazole 33, Pimozide 32, Sulpiride 24, Tiapride 21, Haloperidol 17, Tetrabenazine 9, Ziprasidone 6 and Quetiapine 4.

Therefore, based on the available evidence, experience with the medication and experts' preference, according to the authors Risperidone could be recommended as a first choice agent for the treatment of tics. Risperidone (possibly combined with a selective serotonin reuptake inhibitor) was recommended as a first choice agent also in patients with co-morbid obsessive-compulsive disorder, based on the results of clinical trials. Adverse reactions (especially weight gain and sedation) were identified as the main limitation of this medication. Other medications received a recommendation as well. Aripiprazole was deemed to have 'great potential', especially in treatment-refractory cases, and probably less pronounced risk of severe weight gain. Among first-generation anti-dopaminergic agents, Pimozide was credited with relatively good evidence with a better adverse reaction profile than Haloperidol. It was recommended that the alpha-2 adrenergic agonist Clonidine can be used, especially in the presence of co-morbid attention-deficit and hyperactivity disorder. Finally, Sulpiride and Tiapride were recommended based on the broad clinical experience and favourable adverse effect profile, despite the need for more controlled studies. According to the authors, the other medications mentioned in Table 7.2 could be considered as alternative options, in case of unsatisfactory response to one or more of the above-mentioned agents.

The authors of the ESSTS guidelines formulated a set of indications for the treatment of tics: tics causing subjective discomfort (e.g. pain or injury), tics causing sustained social problems for the patient (e.g. social isolation or bullying), tics causing psychological and emotional problems (e.g. reactive affective symptoms) and tics causing functional interference (e.g. impairment of academic achievements). The ESSTS guidelines did not contain dosage recommendations for each medication. The authors advised that, in general, dosage should start low and gradually increase with close monitoring of both response and adverse reactions. The authors observed that most published studies had included both children and adults, and no evidence suggested that the two age groups should be treated in different ways apart from medication dosages. Moreover, they suggested that the dosage of pharmacotherapy for Tourette syndrome was not different between children, adolescents and adults once body weight had been taken into account, although clear data were lacking.

The authors acknowledged that with most medications (with few exceptions, such as Haloperidol), prescription was based on off-label indications across European countries, reflecting the paucity of efficacy and safety data. It was highlighted that the problem of insufficient data for approval by the registration authority should be discussed with the patients and their families prior to initiation of treatment. Finally, it was suggested that the

Table 7.2 Summary of European and UK (2011) guidelines on the pharmacotherapy of tic disorders

Medication	Additional indication	Starting dose	Therapeutic dose	Level of evidence[a]
First-generation anti-dopaminergic medications				
Haloperidol	–	0.25–0.5 mg	0.25–15 mg	A
Pimozide	–	0.5–1 mg	1–6 mg	A
Second-generation anti-dopaminergic medications				
Aripiprazole	–	2.5 mg	2.5–30 mg	C
Olanzapine	OCB	2.5–5 mg	2.5–20 mg	B
Quetiapine	–	100–150 mg	100–600 mg	C
Risperidone	DBD	0.25 mg	0.25–6 mg	A
Ziprasidone	–	5–10 mg	5–10 mg	A
Alpha-2 adrenergic medications				
Clonidine	ADHD	0.05 mg	0.1–0.3 mg	A
Guanfacine	ADHD	0.5–1 mg	1–4 mg	A
Other tic-suppressing medications				
Sulpiride	OCB	50–100 mg	2–10 mg/kg	B
Tiapride	–	50–100 mg	2–10 mg/kg	B

[a] Evidence Level A (two controlled randomized trials), B (one controlled, randomized trial), C (case studies, open trials).
Abbreviations. ADHD, attention-deficit hyperactivity disorder; DBD disruptive behaviour disorder; OCB obsessive-compulsive behaviour.

treatment of each individual patient should be carefully planned by considering the availablediagnostic information, the level of impairment associated with tics, the efficacy data and adverse reactions of treatment options, as well as the patient's own preference (after psychoeducation), in order to achieve the best result and adherence possible.

Canada (2012)

Two guidelines on the assessment and treatment of Tourette syndrome were published in the Canadian Journal of Psychiatry by the Canadian experts in 2012. The two documents covered the evidence-based pharmacotherapy of tic disorders and the non-pharmacological treatment interventions (behavioural therapy, deep brain stimulation and transcranial magnetic stimulation). The pharmacotherapy guideline sought to provide practising clinicians with guidance on the pharmacological management of tic disorders in children and adults. The authors performed a systematic review of the literature on the treatment of tic disorders, synthesizing the current evidence from studies in both children and adults and providing recommendations based on the evidence while incorporating clinical expertise. Moreover, a multi-institutional group of 14 experts in psychiatry, child psychiatry, neurology, paediatrics and psychology engaged in a consensus meeting. The evidence was presented and discussed, and nominal group techniques were employed to arrive at consensus on recommendations. The consensus group considered the evidence both in children and adults, and recommendations apply to both age groups. When extracting the available evidence, the authors were limited by the strength of the available evidence, as many of the reviewed trials were small, and included clinically heterogeneous samples. The authors also noted that the reviewed studies performed before 1990 used a wide variety of outcome measures for the assessment of tic severity, and frequently used crossover study designs, with poor reporting of results. Therefore the authors stated that they were unable to perform a meta-analysis of study results for most medications. A decrease in the YGTSS total tic score of 8 points (out of 50) was considered clinically meaningful. The authors subsequently graded the body of evidence for each medication as high ('we are very confident that the true effect lies close to that of the estimate of the effect'), moderate ('we are moderately confident in the effect estimate: the true effect is likely to be close to the estimate of the effect, but there is a possibility that it is substantially different'), low ('our confidence in the effect estimate is limited: the true effect may be substantially different from the estimate of the effect') or very low ('we have very little confidence in the effect estimate: the true effect is likely to be substantially different from the estimate of the effect'), according to the Grading of Recommendations, Assessment, Development and Evaluations (GRADE) system. A classification scheme based on the GRADE system was also used to make formal recommendations for the treatment of tics (Table 7.3). A strong recommendation was made when the benefits of treatment clearly outweigh the risks and burdens, and can apply to most patients in most circumstances without reservation. A weak recommendation was made when the benefits, risks and burdens are more closely balanced, and the best action may differ depending on circumstances. The authors also created a third category for medications where insufficient evidence existed to make a formal recommendation.

Based on these principles, strong recommendations were made for the use of Clonidine and Guanfacine (children only) for the treatment of tics. While the evidence supports the efficacy of several anti-dopaminergic medications for the treatment of tics, the high rates of adverse effects associated with these agents resulted in downgrading of recommendations to the weak category. With a weak recommendation, the benefits are closely balanced with the risks and side effects. In situations where tics are not severe or disabling, the use of a medication with only a weak recommendation is not warranted. However, when tics are more distressing and interfering, the need for tic suppression to improve quality of life is stronger, and patients and clinicians may be more willing to accept the risks of pharmacotherapy. The medications with weak recommendations for the treatment of tics included Aripiprazole, Fluphenazine, Haloperidol, Metoclopramide (children only), Olanzapine, Pimozide, Quetiapine, Risperidone, Tetrabenazine, Topiramate and Ziprasidone.

Among the available pharmacological treatment options, the Canadian consensus group determined that Clonidine and Guanfacine should be considered first-line medications for tics, followed by Aripiprazole and Risperidone as second-line medications. Fluphenazine, Haloperidol, Pimozide and Ziprasidone were considered third-line pharmacological options. In young patients with a co-morbid diagnosis of attention-deficit and hyperactivity disorder, the use of Clonidine or Guanfacine for tics was favoured, as evidence supports their efficacy for treating the behavioural co-morbidity as well. For patients who are overweight at baseline, the authors recommended avoiding Olanzapine, Quetiapine and Risperidone because of the risk of further weight gain as an adverse effect of these medications. A further recommendation was that before starting therapy, patients should

Table 7.3 Summary of Canadian (2012) guidelines on the pharmacotherapy of tic disorders

Medication	Dosing suggestions	GRADE recommendations
First-generation anti-dopaminergic medications		
Fluphenazine	0.25–3 mg (children) 2.5–10 mg (adults)	Weak recommendation, low-quality evidence
Haloperidol	0.5–3 mg (children) 0.5–3 mg (adults)	Weak recommendation, high-quality evidence
Pimozide	1–4 mg (children) 1–6 mg (adults)	Weak recommendation, high-quality evidence
Second-generation anti-dopaminergic medications		
Aripiprazole	2–15 mg (children) 2–20 mg (adults)	Weak recommendation, low-quality evidence
Olanzapine	2.5–10 mg (children) 2.5–20 mg (adults)	Weak recommendation, low-quality evidence
Quetiapine	25–400 mg (children) 25–400 mg (adults)	Weak recommendation, very low quality evidence
Risperidone	0.25–3 mg (children) 0.25–6 mg (adults)	Weak recommendation, high-quality evidence
Ziprasidone	20–40 mg (children)	Weak recommendation, low-quality evidence (children)
Alpha-2 adrenergic medications		
Clonidine	0.025–0.3 mg (children) 0.025–0.6 mg (adults)	Strong recommendation, moderate-quality evidence
Guanfacine	0.5–3 mg (children)	Strong recommendation, moderate-quality evidence (children)
Other tic-suppressing medications		
Metoclopramide	0.5 mg/kg, up to 40 mg (children)	Weak recommendation, low-quality evidence (children)
Tetrabenazine	12.5–50 mg (children) 12.5–100 mg (adults)	Weak recommendation, very low quality evidence
Topiramate	1–9 mg/kg (children) 50–200 mg (adults)	Weak recommendation, low-quality evidence

Abbreviations. GRADE, Grading of Recommendations, Assessment, Development and Evaluations.

be informed that medications only suppress their tics in the present and do not alter the natural history of their condition. In consideration of the natural history of tic disorders, the authors stated that medications should be tapered periodically to determine if the treatment is still required. Finally, it was acknowledged that the ability of clinicians to predict which treatment has the greatest chance of success for a given patient is limited.

US (2013)

In 2013, a group of North American experts in Tourette syndrome and the American Academy of Child and Adolescent Psychiatry (AACAP) Committee on Quality Issues produced a Practice Parameter for the assessment and treatment of children and adolescents with tic disorders, published in the Journal of the American Academy of Child and Adolescent Psychiatry. This effort was prompted by the increased complexity in assessing the medical and psychiatric well-being of children presenting with tic disorders and related co-morbid conditions, as well as developments in evidence-based pharmacotherapy and behavioural therapy. The AACAP Practice Parameter was based on a systematic review of the evidence from research and clinical experience in the evaluation and treatment of paediatric tic disorders. The authors explained that the recommendations listed in their comprehensive and developmentally sensitive Parameter are applicable to children, adolescents and young adults. They also acknowledged that although the AACAP Practice Parameter was developed to assist clinicians in psychiatric decision-making, this document was not intended to define the sole standard of care and the ultimate judgement regarding the care of a particular patient must be made by the clinician in light of all of the information presented by the patient (and proxies), the diagnostic and treatment options available, and other relevant resources (Table 7.4).

The AACAP Practice Parameter consists of a set of nine recommendations for best assessment (four recommendations) and treatment practices (five recommendations) of young patients with tic disorders. Each recommendation was presented with the strength of the underlying empirical and/or clinical support, according to one out of four categories. The Clinical Standard category was applied to recommendations based on rigorous empirical evidence (e.g. meta-analyses, systematic reviews, randomized controlled trials) and/or overwhelming clinical consensus. The Clinical Guideline category was applied to recommendations based on strong empirical evidence (e.g. non-randomized controlled trials, cohort studies, case-control studies) and/or strong clinical consensus. The Clinical Option category was applied to recommendations based on emerging empirical evidence (e.g. uncontrolled trials or case series/reports) or clinical opinion, in the absence of strong empirical evidence/consensus. The Not Endorsed category was applied to practices known to be ineffective or contraindicated.

The four recommendations about the assessment of young patients with tic disorders were all presented with Clinical Standard level of support. It was stated that the psychiatric assessment should involve routine screening for unusual movements, stereotypies, tics and family history of tic disorders. If the clinician's screening receives endorsement of the possibility of tics or the clinician observes tics during the evaluation, a more systematic assessment for tic disorders should be conducted. The authors mentioned the age of onset, types of tics, tic frequency, alleviating and aggravating factors, and family history of tics (as well as the possible use of rating scales specific for tics) as part of the more thorough assessment for tics. A separate recommendation reminded that the assessment for new-onset tics or tic-like movements should involve a careful examination for general medical condition or substance aetiologies. It was stated that certain clinical features (e.g. the sudden

Table 7.4 Summary of US (2013) guidelines on the pharmacotherapy of tic disorders

Medication	FDA approval	Starting dose	Therapeutic dose	Main comments
First-generation anti-dopaminergic medications				
Haloperidol	TS	0.25–0.5 mg	1–4 mg	EPS concerns; reports of anxiety flares
Pimozide	TS	0.5–1 mg	2–8 mg	ECG monitoring
Fluphenazine	–	0.5–1 mg	1.5–10 mg	Risk of EPS lower than with Haloperidol
Second-generation anti-dopaminergic medications				
Aripiprazole	–[a]	1–2.5 mg	2.5–15 mg	No prolactin elevation; reports of improvement in OCD
Olanzapine	–	2.5–5 mg	2.5–12.5 mg	Metabolic effects are a major concern
Quetiapine	–	25 mg	25–200 mg	Metabolic effects
Risperidone	–	0.125–0.5 mg	0.75–3 mg	Metabolic effects; prolactin elevation
Ziprasidone	–	5–10 mg	10–40 mg	Current available doses above those used in RCTs
Alpha-2 adrenergic medications				
Clonidine	ADHD	0.025–0.05 mg	0.1–0.4 mg	Sedation, short acting, most helpful for those with initial insomnia
Guanfacine	ADHD	0.5–1 mg	1–4 mg	Support especially for tics + ADHD
Other tic-suppressing medications				
Sulpiride	Not approved in US	50–100 mg	100–500 mg	Larger open-label paediatric study (n = 189)
Tetrabenazine	–	25 mg	37.5–150 mg	Sedation, weight gain, depression
Tiapride	Not approved in US	50–100 mg	2 100–500 mg	–

[a] Aripiprazole was approved by the FDA for the treatment of Tourette syndrome in 2014.
Abbreviations. ADHD, attention-deficit hyperactivity disorder; ECG, electrocardiogram; EPS, extrapyramidal side effects; FDA, Food and Drug Administration; OCD, obsessive-compulsive disorder; RCT, randomized controlled trial.

onset of severe tics, atypical tics or mental status abnormalities suggestive of an organic process) should prompt further medical investigation. Standard blood tests (including full blood count, renal/hepatic function, thyroid function and ferritin level, along with urine drug screen for adolescents) were deemed reasonable. The authors added that in case of abnormally sudden onset or severe symptom exacerbation, the clinician may assess for co-occurring infection with diagnostic tests that indicate acute illness (e.g. culture, rapid viral tests). Electroencephalography and neuroimaging were not routinely recommended and were reserved for cases with other neurological findings. Additional specialty consultation (e.g. paediatric neurology, genetics) was mentioned as possibly helpful in cases with unusual or complex presentations. The final recommendation of the first group stated that the assessment for tic disorders should involve a careful examination for co-morbid psychiatric conditions.

The second group of five recommendations about the treatment of young patients with tic disorders was presented with more heterogeneous levels of support. A recommendation based on Clinical Standard level stated that education regarding chronic tic disorders should be provided, addressing expectations for course and prognosis, and treatment planning should consider classroom-based accommodations. The authors specified that psychoeducation directed at the young patient and family should include common clinical presentations, tic-exacerbating and alleviating factors, risks related to co-morbid conditions, prognosis and treatment options. It was highlighted that parents should be guided to information on tic disorders designed for teachers and school personnel: ignoring of the tics and granting permission to leave the classroom as needed were mentioned as two of the most common forms of accommodation provided by the teachers. A further recommendation based on Clinical Standard level stated that treatment for chronic tic disorders should address the levels of impairment and distress caused by the tics as well as any co-morbid conditions. The authors commented that the decision to treat tics is a sensitive one, made in conjunction with both the child and the family: if the tics are mild in severity, there may be no need for intervention after psychoeducation is provided, as young patients and their families often cope well with tics of mild to moderate severity until pre-teen age years or middle school, at which time teasing from peers may prompt intervention. It was acknowledged that it is often the co-morbid condition, rather than the tic disorder itself, that causes the most severe impairment in functioning or has the most significant impact on quality of life. When establishing the treatment hierarchy, the most impairing condition should be addressed first: as a result, the initial interventions frequently target symptoms from a co-morbid condition, with only ongoing monitoring of tics. The authors added that potential adverse events associated with treatment interventions should be carefully weighed. A recommendation based on Clinical Guideline level stated that behavioural interventions for chronic tic disorders should be considered when tics cause impairment, when they are moderate in severity or if behavioural-responsive psychiatric co-morbidities are present. In addition to addressing behavioural strategies for the treatment of tics (e.g. habit reversal training), the authors commented that behavioural therapy may also address less adaptive coping strategies (e.g. avoidance, withdrawal) that develop secondary to tics and contribute to heightened impairment. Specifically, in some young patients, self-concept can become overly centred on their tics rather than focusing on their areas of strength and resilience: skill-based therapies that target distorted cognitions and avoidance should be beneficial in improving quality of life and reducing sustained reliance on problematic coping mechanisms. A recommendation focusing on the use of pharmacotherapy was based on Clinical

Guideline level. The authors stated that medications for chronic tic disorders should be considered for moderate to severe tics causing severe impairment in quality of life or when medication responsive psychiatric co-morbidities are present that target both tics and co-morbid conditions. In consideration of the existence of a few large, multi-site, randomized, placebo-controlled trials for the treatment of tic disorders, it was argued that pharmacotherapy for tics should have evidence-based support whenever feasible. The authors acknowledged that although the only Food and Drug Administration-approved medications to treat tic disorders were Haloperidol and Pimozide, most clinicians use second-generation anti-dopaminergic medications before first-generation anti-dopaminergic agents, because of concerns about tolerability. Likewise, it was highlighted that some prescribers prefer to use alpha-2 adrenergic agonists as first-line agents over anti-dopaminergic medications because of the better adverse effect profile, combined with an estimated effect size of 0.5 for the amelioration of tics.

The authors added a few comments on the treatment in context of co-morbidity. With regard to co-morbid obsessive-compulsive disorder, since some studies suggested that the presence of tics may yield a less robust response to selective serotonin reuptake inhibitors, it was noted that the use of an anti-dopaminergic medication as augmentation therapy may result in additional benefit for young patients with both tics and obsessive-compulsive symptoms. With regard to co-morbid attention-deficit and hyperactivity disorder, the authors acknowledged previous concerns of worsening tic severity with the use of central nervous system stimulants, reflected in the Food and Drug Administration package insert listing tics as a contraindication for these medications. However they highlighted that for young patients with co-morbid attention-deficit and hyperactivity disorder, new evidence demonstrated that tics are not universally increased by stimulant medication, although the presence of tics appeared to limit the maximum dose achieved. With regard to co-morbid anxiety and affective disorders, the authors suggested that, in the absence of dedicated studies in patients with tic disorders, the best approach was to use evidence-based treatment for anxiety and affective conditions. It was also noted that disruptive behaviour disorder (including explosive anger and rage outbursts) was shown to be relatively common among young patients with tics, affecting up to 80 per cent of patients in specialist clinics. The authors acknowledged the lack of controlled pharmacological studies in young patients with tic disorders and aggressive/anger outbursts, and suggested that behavioural therapies addressing antecedents (including sensory issues and poor frustration tolerance) and anger management may be useful. Preliminary positive findings for second-generation anti-dopaminergic agents, as well as for selective serotonin reuptake inhibitors, were interpreted cautiously in consideration of the significant design limitations, small samples, relatively weak effects and associated risks. According to the final recommendation (Not Endorsed category), deep brain stimulation, repetitive magnetic stimulation, special diets and dietary supplements lack empirical support for the treatment of Tourette syndrome and other tic disorders and are not recommended.

UK (2016)

In 2016 a group of experts based in the UK published a health technology assessment on the clinical effectiveness and patient perspectives of different treatment strategies for tics in children and adolescents with Tourette syndrome. This document contained two parts, combining the results of a systematic review and a qualitative analysis, which had been previously presented in two articles published in 2016 and in 2015 in the *Journal of Child Psychology and Psychiatry* and in *BMC Psychiatry*, respectively.

Part I consisted in a systematic review and meta-analysis of the benefits and risks of pharmacological, behavioural and physical interventions for tics in children and adolescents with Tourette syndrome or other chronic tic disorders. The critical outcome for the systematic review was tic severity/frequency, and the authors also included studies in adults or mixed populations, which were considered as supporting evidence. The Cochrane risk of bias tool was used for the risk of bias assessment and the GRADE approach for assessing the overall quality of the evidence was included in the quantitative systematic review (70 studies out a total of 6345 citations screened). For outcomes measuring benefit of treatment, the authors used the standardized mean difference (SMD) as the effect size, calculated as the difference in mean change scores divided by the pooled standard deviation of the change scores. The SMD was standardized so that a negative effect size indicated that the outcome favoured the intervention relative to the control (Table 7.5).

The findings of this systematic review and evidence synthesis showed that there are effective medications (e.g. anti-dopaminergic agents and alpha-2 adrenergic agonists) available for the treatment of tics in children and adolescents with Tourette syndrome. However, the number and quality of the existing clinical trials was low, resulting in downgrading of the strength of both the evidence and conclusions. The need for larger and better-conducted trials addressing important clinical uncertainties was acknowledged. The authors concluded that when medication is considered appropriate for the treatment of tics, the balance of clinical benefits to harm favours alpha-2 adrenergic agonists (Clonidine and Guanfacine) as first-line options. Anti-dopaminergic agents were regarded as likely to be useful as second-line options (when alpha-2 adrenergic agonists are either ineffective or poorly tolerated), in consideration of their tolerability profiles. Specifically, despite the quality of the evidence was generally low, the main review findings suggested that there is clear evidence that both anti-dopaminergic agents and alpha-2 adrenergic agonists produce improvements in tics that may be clinically meaningful in children and adolescents with Tourette syndrome. Moreover, the available evidence suggested that clinically significant differences in tic reduction between anti-dopaminergic agents and alpha-2 adrenergic agonists are unlikely. There was no clear evidence that the clinical effectiveness of medications belonging to these pharmacological classes is moderated by either tic severity or co-morbidity. Both Metoclopramide and Topiramate were included among other agents with evidence suggesting effectiveness in reducing tics. However, the authors added that the known adverse effect profiles of these medications, balanced against relatively weak and poor-quality evidence of benefits, meant that these agents are unlikely to be considered clinically useful for treating tics. Finally, there was very low quality evidence that medications used to treat co-morbid obsessive-compulsive disorder and attention-deficit and hyperactivity disorder (selective serotonin reuptake inhibitors and central nervous system stimulants/atomoxetine, respectively) significantly exacerbate or worsen tics in the short term.

Part II consisted in a qualitative study to explore the experience of services and treatment and to understand which outcomes are most valued from the perspective of young patients with Tourette syndrome and parents of young patients with Tourette syndrome. In addition to a qualitative systematic review of four studies, data were collected from two sources: an online national survey of the experiences of care and treatment of 358 parents of children and adolescents with Tourette syndrome, and a series of in-depth qualitative interviews with 40 young patients with Tourette syndrome (median age 13 years; age range 11–17 years) to

Table 7.5 Summary of UK (2016) guidelines on the pharmacotherapy of tic disorders

Medication	Age group	Benefit (SMD and 95% CI)	Certainty in the effect estimate (GRADE)
First-generation anti-dopaminergic medications			
Haloperidol	Children + adults	−0.50 (−0.89, −0.10)	Low (downgraded because of suboptimal sample size and high risk of bias)
Pimozide	Children	−0.81 (−1.24, −0.38)	Low (downgraded because of suboptimal sample size and high risk of bias)
Second-generation anti-dopaminergic medications			
Aripiprazole	Children	−0.62 (−1.14, −0.11)	Moderate (downgraded because of suboptimal sample size)
Risperidone	Children	−1.18 (−2.02, −0.34)	Low (downgraded because of suboptimal sample size)
Ziprasidone	Children	−0.74 (−1.54, 0.06)	Low (downgraded because of suboptimal sample size and high risk of bias)
Alpha-2 adrenergic medications			
Clonidine/ Guanfacine	Children	−0.74 (−1.06, −0.42)	Moderate (downgraded because of suboptimal sample size)
Other tic-suppressing medications			
Metoclopramide	Children	−1.43 (−2.28, −0.59)	Moderate (downgraded because of suboptimal sample size and high risk of bias)
Topiramate	Children + adults	−0.88 (−1.68, −0.08)	Low (downgraded because of suboptimal sample size)

Abbreviations. CI, confidence interval; GRADE, Grading of Recommendations, Assessment, Development and Evaluations; SMD, standardized mean difference.

explore their experiences of care and treatment. Useful data were analysed from 295 respondents (of which 92.2 per cent were mothers) to the online survey hosted via the Tourettes Action–UK website. Interview transcripts were evaluated using thematic analysis and responses to survey open-ended questions were assessed using content analysis. Triangulation of qualitative and quantitative data from the parents' survey and qualitative data from the interviews with young patients were used to increase the validity and depth of the findings. The main results of the online national survey showed that just over half of young patients with Tourette syndrome had received medication for tics. The most commonly used drugs were Aripiprazole, Clonidine and Risperidone. Both young patients and parents reported that medication could be helpful in reducing tics, but frequently expressed concerns about adverse effects and lack of provision of relevant information explaining the rationale for using medication for tics and possible adverse effects. The parents of young patients with Tourette syndrome perceived Aripiprazole as being most helpful for tic control with least troublesome adverse effects. While regarding reduction of the frequency and intensity of tics and increased control over tics as the most important treatment outcomes, young patients with Tourette syndrome (and – to a lesser extent – parents) highlighted the importance of recognizing and managing anxiety symptoms and stress associated with tics. In addition to the importance of reducing anxiety and emotional symptoms in Tourette syndrome, other key themes from the qualitative study included difficulties in access to specialist care and delay in diagnosis (an average of 3 years from onset of tics). Lack of information on dosing and comparison with a control intervention means that findings in the qualitative study relating to the experience of treatment could not be interpreted as evidence of effectiveness or lack of harm.

US (2019)

A multidisciplinary panel convened by the American Academy of Neurology (AAN) guideline committee performed a systematic review and developed guideline recommendations on the assessment and treatment of tics in both children and adults with Tourette syndrome and other chronic tic disorders. Both the systematic literature review and the set of recommendations were published in the journal *Neurology* in 2019. The literature review for this practice guideline systematically evaluated the efficacy of treatments for tics and the risks associated with their use. In line with the methodological practice recommended by the AAN, the authors assessed systematic reviews and randomized controlled trials on the treatment of tics that included at least 20 participants (10 participants if a crossover trial). The authors calculated the effect size, expressed as a measure of the size of the intervention effect relative to the variability observed in each study (SMD). For their analysis, an SMD of 0.20 was considered the minimal clinically meaningful difference for reduction in tic severity, whereas effect sizes smaller than 0.10 were considered clinically unimportant (Table 7.6). There was moderate confidence that a few of the most commonly used medications for tics, including Aripiprazole, Clonidine, Haloperidol, Risperidone and Tiapride, were probably more likely than placebo to reduce tics. There was low confidence that other commonly used agents, such as Guanfacine, Metoclopramide, Pimozide, Topiramate and Ziprasidone, were possibly more likely than placebo to reduce tics. The authors acknowledged that while they found evidence to support the efficacy of several treatments, many of the interventions had only been studied in one randomized controlled trial of short duration, with modest sample sizes.

In 2016, the Guideline Development, Dissemination, and Implementation Subcommittee of the AAN recruited a multidisciplinary panel to develop guideline recommendations on the assessment and treatment of tics, including nine physicians, two psychologists and two patient representatives associated with the Tourette Association of America. This evidence-based practice guideline followed the methodologies described in the 2011 edition of the AAN's guideline development process manual, as amended to include use of the revised scheme for classifying therapeutic articles and the change in order of steps for external review. The evidence-based conclusions from the systematic review formed the foundation of the AAN process, but other factors influenced the structure of the guideline. Specifically, the practice recommendations included in the guideline were supported by structured justifications, integrating evidence from the systematic review and

Table 7.6 Summary of US (2019) guidelines on the pharmacotherapy of tic disorders

Medication	Age group	Benefit (SMD and 95% CI)	Certainty in the effect estimate (GRADE)
First-generation anti-dopaminergic medications			
Haloperidol	Children + adults	0.59 (0.11, 1.06)	Moderate (two Class II studies)
Pimozide	Children + adults	0.66 (0.06, 1.25)	Low (three Class II studies – confidence in evidence downgraded due to imprecision)
Second-generation anti-dopaminergic medications			
Aripiprazole	Children	0.64 (0.31, −0.97)	Moderate (one Class I study)
Risperidone	Children + adults	0.79 (0.31, 1.27)	Moderate (two Class II studies)
Ziprasidone	Children	1.14 (0.32, 1.97)	Low (one Class II study)
Alpha-2 adrenergic medications			
Clonidine	Children + adults	0.45 (0.13, 0.77)	Moderate (one Class I study + two Class II studies)
Guanfacine	Children	0.45 (0.03, 0.87)	Low (one Class I study + two Class II studies – confidence in evidence downgraded due to imprecision)
Other tic-suppressing medications			
Metoclopramide	Children	1.14 (0.33, 1.95)	Low (one Class II study)
Tiapride	Children	0.62 (0.36, 0.88)	Moderate (one Class I study)
Topiramate	Children + adults	0.91 (0.11, 1.71)	Low (one Class I study)

Abbreviations. CI, confidence interval; GRADE, Grading of Recommendations, Assessment, Development and Evaluations; SMD, standardized mean difference.

other sources. In the resulting practice guideline, the limitations of the currently available evidence were acknowledged, and psychoeducation and shared decision-making regarding treatment needs and priorities were strongly encouraged. The authors explicitly addressed the question of when clinicians and patients should pursue treatment for tics, as well as the question of how clinicians and patients should choose between evidence-based treatment options and determine the sequence or combinations of treatments.

A total of 46 recommendations were formulated regarding the assessment and management of tics in children and adults with Tourette syndrome and other chronic tic disorders. In addition to pharmacotherapy, the topics included counselling recommendations on the natural history of tic disorders, psychoeducation for teachers and peers, assessment for co-morbid conditions and periodic re-assessment of the need for ongoing therapy. The authors highlighted that treatment options should be individualized, and the choice should be the result of a collaborative decision process involving patients, caregivers and clinicians. As part of this process, the benefits and harms of individual treatments, as well as the presence of co-morbid disorders, were taken into account. Watchful waiting was included in the treatment options, and recommendations were provided on how to offer and monitor different therapies, including medications.

Each recommendation was justified by deductive arguments that were documented, in a transparent manner, by four types of premises (rationale statements): evidence-based conclusions from the systematic review, generally accepted principles of care, strong evidence from related conditions and deductive inferences from other premises. When sufficient evidence supported an inference for the use of an intervention (i.e. the balance of benefits and harms favoured the intervention), the development panel assigned one of three designations, denoting the level of strength of the recommendation. Level A was associated with the strongest recommendation level: these recommendations, denoted by the use of the verb 'must', were rare because they are based on high confidence in the evidence and require both a high magnitude of benefit and low risk. Level B corresponded to the verb 'should': these recommendations were more common because the requirements were less stringent, albeit still based on the evidence and benefit-risk profile. Level C corresponded to the verb 'may': the lowest allowable recommendation considered useful by the AAN within the scope of clinical practice, accommodating the highest degree of practice variation. Finally, a few key non-evidence-based factors were transparently and systematically considered when formulating the recommendations: the relative value of the benefit compared with the risk, the feasibility of complying with the intervention (e.g. because of its availability), the cost of the intervention and the expected variation in patient preferences relative to the risks, burdens and benefits of the intervention.

It was noted that providing information to families about the natural history of a disorder can help inform treatment decisions (although there was no evidence that treatment was more effective the earlier it was started). In line with this principle, two Level A recommendations were formulated: clinicians must inform patients and their caregivers about the natural history of tic disorders and evaluate functional impairment related to tics from the perspective of the patient and, if applicable, the caregiver. Moreover, as a result of partial or complete remission during the natural course of the disorder, medication prescribed for tics in young patients may no longer be required over time. A further Level A recommendation stated that physicians prescribing medications for tics must periodically re-evaluate the need for ongoing medical treatment. As the natural history of Tourette syndrome suggested that tics may improve with time, a Level B recommendation was formulated, stating that clinicians should inform patients and caregivers that watchful waiting is an acceptable approach in patients who do not experience functional impairment from their tics.

Strong evidence from related conditions indicated that psychoeducation about Tourette syndrome with peers can result in more positive attitudes towards patients, while psychoeducation with teachers can improve knowledge about the condition. It was therefore inferred that improving peers' attitudes about and teachers' knowledge of Tourette syndrome may positively affect patients. A Level B recommendation stated that clinicians should refer patients with Tourette syndrome to resources for psychoeducation for teachers and peers, such as the Tourette Association of America. The authors of the AAN guideline inferred from the existing evidence that use of validated scales to measure tic severity (e.g. the YGTSS) can aid the evaluation of treatment response in the clinical setting. This resulted in a Level C recommendation that clinicians may measure tic severity using a valid scale to assess treatment effects. According to an evidence-base Level A recommendation, clinicians must counsel patients that treatments for tics, including medications, infrequently result in complete cessation of tics (Level A).

Evidence from trials mainly conducted in children indicated that patients with tics receiving alpha-2 adrenergic agonists are probably (Clonidine) or possibly (Guanfacine) more likely than those receiving placebo to have reduced tic severity. Moreover, in children with tics and co-morbid attention-deficit and hyperactivity disorder, Clonidine and Guanfacine demonstrated beneficial effects on both tics and attention-deficit and hyperactivity symptoms: in fact, the effect size of these medications on tics appeared larger in children with tics and attention-deficit and hyperactivity disorder compared with patients with tics without a co-morbid diagnosis of attention-deficit and hyperactivity disorder. Based on these findings, the AAN guideline included a Level B recommendation according to which clinicians should counsel patients with tics and co-morbid attention-deficit and hyperactivity disorder that alpha-2 adrenergic agonists may provide benefit for both conditions. With regard to adverse effects, there was evidence that, relative to placebo, Clonidine is probably associated with higher rates of sedation, and Guanfacine is probably associated with higher rates of drowsiness. There was evidence from studies in young patients with attention-deficit and hyperactivity disorder that alpha-2 adrenergic agonists can cause hypotension, bradycardia, sedation (both Clonidine and Guanfacine) and QTc prolongation (Guanfacine extended release), whereas their abrupt withdrawal may cause rebound hypertension. This body of evidence was in line with one Level B recommendation (clinicians should prescribe alpha-2 adrenergic agonists for the treatment of tics when the benefits of treatment outweigh the risks) and four Level A recommendations: clinicians must counsel patients with tics regarding the adverse effects of alpha-2 adrenergic agonists (including sedation); clinicians must monitor heart rate and blood pressure (plus QTc interval in patients on Guanfacine extended release with a history of cardiac conditions, patients taking other QT-prolonging agents, or patients with a family history of long QT syndrome); clinicians discontinuing alpha-2 adrenergic agonists must gradually taper them to avoid rebound hypertension.

With regard to anti-dopaminergic medications, there was evidence that Aripiprazole, Haloperidol, Risperidone and Tiapride are probably more likely than placebo to reduce tic severity, whereas Metoclopramide, Pimozide and Ziprasidone are possibly more likely than placebo to reduce tic severity. There was insufficient evidence to determine the relative efficacy of these medications. Systematic reviews of trials and cohort studies demonstrated a higher risk of medication-induced movement disorders (including acute dystonia, akathisia, drug-induced parkinsonism, tardive dyskinesia and tardive dystonia), metabolic adverse effects, weight gain, prolactin increase and QT prolongation with both first and second-generation anti-dopaminergic medications across psychiatric and neurological conditions. Specifically, the long-term use of Metoclopramide was associated with tardive dyskinesia, resulting in a black box warning from the Food and Drug Administration. Relative to placebo, the evidence from studies in patients with tics demonstrated a higher risk of medication-induced movement disorders with Haloperidol, Pimozide and Risperidone; a higher risk of weight gain with Aripiprazole and Risperidone; a higher risk of somnolence with Aripiprazole, Risperidone and Tiapride; a higher risk of QT prolongation with Pimozide; and a higher risk of elevated prolactin with Haloperidol, Metoclopramide and Pimozide. The relative propensity for each adverse effect was found to vary by medication and was often dose-dependent. These lines of evidence on the efficacy and tolerability of anti-dopaminergic medications resulted in one Level C recommendation (clinicians may prescribe anti-dopaminergic medications for the treatment of tics when the benefits of treatment outweigh the risks) and two Level A recommendations: clinicians must counsel patients on the relative propensity of anti-dopaminergic medications for extrapyramidal, metabolic and hormonal adverse effects to inform decision-making on which anti-dopaminergic agent should be prescribed; clinicians must also prescribe the lowest effective dose of anti-dopaminergic medication for tics to decrease the risk of adverse effects. Moreover, a Level B recommendation stated that clinicians prescribing anti-dopaminergic medications for tics should monitor for medication-induced movement disorders and for metabolic and hormonal adverse effects of anti-dopaminergic agents, using evidence-based monitoring protocols. According to a Level A recommendation, clinicians prescribing anti-dopaminergic medications for tics must perform electrocardiography and measure the QTc interval before and after starting Pimozide or Ziprasidone, or if the anti-dopaminergic agents are co-administered with other medications that can prolong the QTc interval. Finally, a Level B recommendation stated that when attempting to discontinue anti-dopaminergic medications for tics, clinicians should gradually taper medications over weeks to months to avoid withdrawal dyskinesias.

In patients with mild but troublesome tics who are not obtaining a satisfactory response or experience adverse effects from other treatments, Topiramate was identified as a potentially useful alternative. A Level B recommendation reported that clinicians should prescribe Topiramate for the treatment of tics when the benefits of treatment outweigh the risks, based on the evidence that this medication is possibly more likely than placebo to reduce tic severity. It was noted that, while generally well tolerated at low doses (25–150 mg/day), Topiramate may cause adverse effects, including cognitive problems (especially word finding difficulties), somnolence and weight loss and may increase the risk of kidney stones. This information was reflected in a Level A recommendation, stating that clinicians must counsel patients regarding common adverse effects of Topiramate, including cognitive and language problems, somnolence, weight loss and an increased risk of kidney stones

A few recommendations were relevant to patients with tics and co-morbid behavioural problems. According to a Level B recommendation, clinicians should ensure an assessment for co-morbid obsessive-compulsive disorder and attention-deficit and hyperactivity disorder is performed in patients with tics, evaluating the burden/functional impairment of behavioural symptoms and ensuring that appropriate treatment is provided. Specifically, the role of cognitive behavioural therapy as first-line intervention for co-morbid obsessive-compulsive disorder was highlighted. In children with tics and attention-deficit and hyperactivity disorder, Clonidine (with or without concomitant use of psychostimulants) and Guanfacine were considered probably more likely than placebo to reduce tic severity and reduce attention-deficit and hyperactivity symptoms. It was observed that while attention-deficit and hyperactivity symptoms may improve in adolescence, adults with Tourette syndrome may require ongoing care for this behavioural co-morbidity.

Both population-based and clinic-based studies showed that patients with Tourette syndrome are at high risk of other psychiatric co-morbidities, including anxiety disorders, affective disorders and disruptive behaviour disorders. Co-morbid affective disorders appeared more prevalent in adolescents and adults than children and in patients with greater tic severity. According to a Level A recommendation, clinicians must ensure appropriate screening for anxiety, affective and disruptive behaviour disorders is performed in patients with tics. Moreover, registry data showed an increased risk of dying by suicide and attempting suicide in patients with Tourette syndrome compared with controls, which persisted after adjusting for psychiatric co-morbidity. Persistence of tics beyond young adulthood, previous suicide attempts and co-morbid personality disorders were found to increase the risk of death by suicide. These observations resulted in a further Level A recommendation stating that clinicians must inquire about suicidal thoughts and suicide attempts in patients with Tourette syndrome and refer to appropriate resources if present.

Guidelines Based on Expert Survey and Consensus

Europe and UK (2012)

In order to systematically examine treatment practices in Tourette syndrome across Europe-based clinicians, all ESSTS members actively prescribing for paediatric and/or adult patients with Tourette syndrome were invited to complete an online questionnaire covering pharmacological treatment of five symptom domains: tics, attention-deficit and hyperactivity symptoms, obsessive-compulsive symptoms, anxiety and depression. The results the first large-scale survey on prescribing habits for the pharmacological management of Tourette syndrome in Europe were published in the European Journal of Paediatric Neurology in 2012.

Out of a total of 86 ESSTS members initially contacted in 2010, 57 clinicians who were actively prescribing for patients with Tourette syndrome were included in the survey. Response rates were good (77 per cent), with 44 clinicians from 18 European countries returning the questionnaire. Only 32 clinicians (73 per cent) provided data on their current occupations. The pool of the responders included 23 psychiatrists (and neuropsychiatrists) and 9 neurologists (and behavioural neurologists); 6 worked with children and adolescents and 26 with adults. According to them, medication choices were predominately determined by the scientific literature ($n = 17$) and previous experience ($n = 17$). The main factor determining whether or not clinicians would start prescribing medications was whether the patient's symptoms caused impairment in their function/development ($n = 26$). In non-urgent circumstances and in between dose changes, clinicians would take 2–4 weeks to titrate the dosages of medications for tics ($n = 13$) and would continue on therapeutic doses for up to 6 weeks before considering medication review, in case of unsatisfactory efficacy of the first-line medication ($n = 22$). The majority of participants (60.5 per cent) did not ask their patients to temporarily stop their medication for specific periods of time, such as summer holidays (sometimes referred to as 'drug holidays').

With regard to medication choice, the results revealed a variety of different agents being prescribed as first-line options. Overall, anti-dopaminergic medications were widely used, and Risperidone was the most commonly prescribed medication for the treatment of tics. However, there was a large variability in both the medication choices and dosages. Finally, with regard to specialists' background, psychiatrists more often prescribed Risperidone as first-line options for tics, whereas neurologists chose Clonidine. In general, clinicians prescribing for children and clinicians prescribing for adults opted for similar pharmacological classes, although their individual medication choices were different. Interestingly, most clinicians working with adults (41.7 per cent) opted for Aripiprazole as first-line option for the treatment of tics, despite the lack of evidence from double-blind controlled

Table 8.1 Top three first-line medication choices for the treatment of tics according to the European Society for the Study of Tourette Syndrome (ESSTS) survey (2012)

Medication	Average starting dose (range)	Average maximum dose (range)
Children (n = 20)		
1. Risperidone	0.5 mg (0.25–1 mg)	2 mg (1–4 mg)
2. Clonidine	0.025 mg (0.025–0.025 mg)	0.1 mg (0.05–0.2 mg)
3. Aripiprazole	2–2.5 mg (0.5–10 mg)	15 mg (4–15 mg)
Adults (n = 12)		
1. Aripiprazole	5 mg (2.5–10 mg)	15 mg (10–30 mg)
2. Risperidone	0.5 mg (0.5–1 mg)	3–4 mg (1–10 mg)
3. Sulpiride	100 mg (100–200 mg)	400–600 mg (400–1400 mg)

trials at the time of the survey (Table 8.1). It is possible that their choice was related to the perception of more favourable tolerability profile for Aripiprazole compared to other anti-dopaminergic agents.

Established pharmacotherapy for tics, such as Haloperidol, Pimozide or Tetrabenazine, were not listed in the top three most commonly prescribed medications for either children or adults with Tourette syndrome. Importantly, the results of the ESSTS survey contradicted previous findings that first-generation anti-dopaminergic medications were the most commonly prescribed agents for the treatment of tics, indicating that there had been a change in prescribing practices over the previous years.

Japan (2019)

A questionnaire-based survey modelled on the 2012 ESSTS survey was conducted in Japan with the aim to collate the consensus of Japanese experts and clarify the current status of pharmacotherapy for tic disorders and co-morbid conditions. The results, published in the journal *Brain and Development* in 2019, were compared with the recent international evidence to improve the quality of pharmacological treatment for tic disorders and co-morbid conditions in Japan. The authors conducted a two-step survey: consultation of national experts with a newly developed questionnaire in the first step; revision and circulation of the modified questionnaire back with feedback of the findings from the first survey in the second step. As part of the initial survey (performed in 2015), the authors devised a questionnaire referring to the ESSTS guidelines (2011) and expert consensus (2012) on pharmacotherapy for patients with Tourette syndrome. The clinicians were members of the Japanese Society of Tourette Syndrome Research (n = 71) or had published research articles on tic disorders or childhood obsessive-compulsive disorder during the 5-year period preceding the survey (n = 52). The questionnaires were received by 115 clinicians, out of whom 54 (46.9 per cent) responded. Of the 54 clinicians who took part in the first step of the survey, 53 were psychiatrists or child specialists: 10 (18.5 per cent) were psychiatrists, 17 (31.5 per cent) child psychiatrists, 23 (42.6 per cent) paediatricians and 3 (5.6 per cent) child neurologists.

The results of the first survey revealed variability in preferred medications and dosages among the experts in Japan. After the first survey, the authors revised the questionnaire to determine the extent of agreement among the experts by using the Delphi method. As part of the second step of the survey (performed in 2016), the revised version of the questionnaire was sent to 30 clinicians. Of the 24 clinicians who took part in the second step of the survey, 4 (16.7 per cent) were psychiatrists, 6 (25.0 per cent) child psychiatrists, 12 (50.0 per cent) paediatricians and 1 (4.2 per cent) was a child neurologist. The authors were able to build a general consensus on pharmacotherapy for tic disorders and co-morbid conditions based on the second survey.

Aripiprazole and Risperidone were identified by the Japanese experts as first- and second-line pharmacological options for tic disorders, respectively (Table 8.2).

Table 8.2 Preferred medications for tics by Japanese experts (2019)

Medication	Children (n = 22)	Older adolescents and adults (n = 22)
Aripiprazole as first choice	20 (90.9%)	20 (90.9%)
Risperidone as first choice	15 (68.2%)	15 (68.2%)
Risperidone as second choice	19 (86.4%)	20 (90.9%)
Haloperidol as second choice	8 (36.4%)	6 (27.3%)

The most important factor in deciding to start pharmacotherapy in children with tic disorders was functional impairment caused by tic symptoms. The age at first prescription of pharmacotherapy for tics was below 6 years for 68.2 per cent of clinicians. Medication dosages were increased after 2 or 4 weeks at the same dose by 76.2 per cent of clinicians and 86.4 per cent of clinicians, respectively; according to 86.4 per cent of clinicians, the main reason for dosage increase was unsatisfactory effectiveness on tic control. In children, Aripiprazole was found to be the first-line medication (90.9 per cent of clinicians). The preferred starting dose of Aripiprazole was 1.5 mg or 3.0 mg (66.7 per cent and 71.4 per cent of clinicians, respectively). Although the preferred maximum doses were 6 mg and 12 mg in the first step of the survey, the level of agreement on this point was insufficient in the second step.

The most important factor in deciding to start pharmacotherapy in older adolescents and adults with tic disorders was functional impairment caused by tic symptoms. Medication dosages were increased after 2 or 4 weeks at the same dose by 68.2 per cent and 86.4 per cent of the clinicians, respectively, and the main reason for the dosage increase was tics continuing without change (90.9 per cent of clinicians). Aripiprazole was considered the first-line medication for tic disorders in older adolescents and adults by most clinicians (90.9 per cent), with Risperidone being the most common second-line option (90.9 per cent of clinicians). The preferred starting dose of Aripiprazole was 3.0 mg (85.7 per cent of clinicians), and the preferred maximum dose was 12 mg or 24 mg (42.9 per cent and 47.6 per cent of clinicians, respectively). The preferred starting dose of Risperidone was 1 mg (77.3 per cent of clinicians), and the preferred maximum dose was 3 mg or 6 mg (36.4 per cent and 20.9 per cent of clinicians, respectively). Alpha-2 adrenergic agonists were prescribed less frequently by Japanese experts, despite their widespread use in the treatment of tic disorders internationally. There were no significant group differences between psychiatrists and paediatricians in the selection of medications or their starting and maximum doses. The authors acknowledged the presence of considerable selection bias, since their final respondents were only 24 clinicians, 21 per cent of the clinicians who initially received the first questionnaires. However, this survey reflected the trends of Japanese experts and identified a widespread consensus on the use of the second-generation anti-dopaminergic medications Aripiprazole and Risperidone for the treatment of tics.

Further reading

The scientific literature on Tourette syndrome has expanded considerably since the new millennium (Figure 9.1).

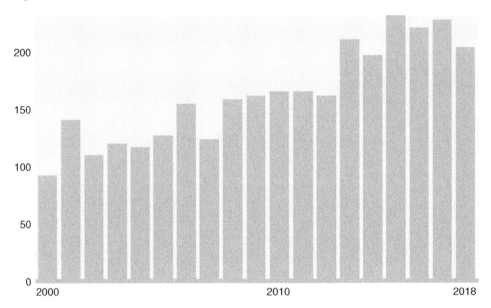

Figure 9.1 Scientific articles on Tourette syndrome indexed in PubMed, 2000–18.

The reference list that closes this handbook is but the tip of the iceberg of scientific contributions on tic disorders and their treatment. Among inevitable omissions, it encompasses relevant articles (sorted by topic), scientific journal issues dedicated to Tourette syndrome and other tic disorders, books on Tourette syndrome and websites containing useful information for both clinicians and patients.

Articles

General Overviews

Bloch M, State M, Pittenger C. Recent advances in Tourette syndrome. Curr Opin Neurol 2011;24:119–25.

Cavanna AE. Gilles de la Tourette syndrome. Neuropsychiatr News 2014;9:17–22.

Cavanna AE, Seri S. Tourette's syndrome. Br Med J 2013;347:f4964.

Cavanna AE, Shah S. Update on Tourette syndrome. Psychiatr Times 2010;27:32–4.

Cavanna AE, Termine C. Tourette syndrome. Adv Exp Med Biol 2012;724:375–83.

Coffey BJ, Biederman J, Geller DA, Spencer T, Park KS, Shapiro SJ, Garfield SB. The course of Tourette's disorder: A literature review. Harvard Rev Psychiatr 2000;8:192–8.

Dooley JM. Tic disorders in childhood. Semin Pediatr Neurol 2006;13:231–42.

Du J-C, Chiu T-F, Lee K-M, Wu H-L, Yang Y-C, Hsu S-Y, Sun C-S, Hwang B, Leckman JF. Tourette syndrome in children: An updated review. Pediatr Neonatol 2010;51:255–64.

Efron D, Dale RC. Tics and Tourette syndrome. J Paediatr Child Health 2018;54:1148–53.

Galvez-Jimenez N. Tics and Tourette syndrome: An adult perspective. Cleve Clin J Med 2012;79(Suppl 2):S35–9.

Ganos C, Martino D. Tics and Tourette syndrome. Neurol Clin 2015;33:115–36.

Ganos C, Munchau A, Bhatia KP. The semiology of tics, Tourette's, and their associations. Mov Disord Clin Pract 2014;1:145–53.

Gilles de la Tourette G. Étude sur une affection nerveuse caractérisée par de l'incoordination motrice accompagnée d'écholalie et de coprolalie. Arch Neurol 1885;9:19–42, 158–200.

Gravino G. Gilles de la Tourette syndrome. Ann Clin Psychiatr 2013;25:297–306.

Gunduz A, Okun MS. A review and update on Tourette syndrome: Where is the field heading? Curr Neurol Neurosci Rep 2016;16:37.

Hallett M. Tourette syndrome: Update. Brain Dev 2015;37:651–5.

Hartmann A, Worbe Y. Tourette syndrome: Clinical spectrum, mechanisms and personalized treatments. Curr Opin Neurol 2018;31:504–9.

Hassan N, Cavanna AE. The prognosis of Tourette syndrome: Implications for clinical practice. Funct Neurol 2012;27:23–7.

Hirschtritt ME, Dy ME, Yang KG, Scharf JM. Diagnosis and treatment of Tourette syndrome. Neurology 2016;87:e65–7.

Itard JMG. Mémoire sur quelques fonctions involontaires des appareils de la locomotion de la préhension et de la voix. Arch Gen Med 1825;8:385–407.

Jankovic J, Kurlan R. Tourette syndrome: Evolving concepts. Mov Disord 2011;26:1149–56.

Jankovic J. Tourette's syndrome. N Engl J Med 2001;345:1184–92.

Kenney C, Kuo SH, Jimenez-Shahed J. Tourette's syndrome. Am Fam Physician 2008;77:651–8.

Leckman JF. Tourette's syndrome. Lancet 2002;360:1577–86.

Martino D, Ganos C, Pringsheim TM. Tourette syndrome and chronic tic disorders: The clinical spectrum beyond tics. Int Rev Neurobiol 2017;134:1461–90.

McNaught KS, Mink JW. Advances in understanding and treatment of Tourette syndrome. Nat Rev Neurol 2011;7:667–76.

Ong MT, Mordekar SR, Seal A. 15 minute consultation: tics and Tourette syndrome. Arch Dis Child Educ Pract Ed 2016;101:87–94.

Plessen KJ. Tic disorders and Tourette's syndrome. Eur Child Adolesc Psychiatr 2013;22(Suppl 1):S55–60.

Pringsheim T. Tourette syndrome and other tic disorders of childhood. Handb Clin Neurol 2013;112:853–6.

Rickards H, Woolf I, Cavanna AE. Trousseau's disease: a description of Gilles de la Tourette syndrome 12 years before 1885. Mov Disord 2010;25:2285–9.

Rickards H. Tourette's syndrome and other tic disorders. Pract Neurol 2010;10:252–9.

Rivera-Navarro J, Cubo E, Almazán J. The diagnosis of Tourette's syndrome: Communication and impact. Clin Child Psychol Psychiatr 2009;14:13–23.

Robertson MM, Eapen V, Singer HS, Martino D, Scharf JM, Paschou P, Roessner V, Woods DW, Hariz M, Mathews CA, Crncec R, Leckman JF. Gilles de la Tourette syndrome. Nature Rev Dis Primers 2017;3:16097.

Robertson MM. A personal 35 year perspective on Gilles de la Tourette syndrome: Prevalence, phenomenology, comorbidities, and coexistent psychopathologies. Lancet Psychiatr 2015;2:68–87.

Robertson MM. A personal 35 year perspective on Gilles de la Tourette syndrome: Assessment, investigations, and management. Lancet Psychiatr 2015;2:88–104.

Robertson MM. Gilles de la Tourette syndrome: The complexities of phenotype and treatment. Br J Hosp Med 2011;72:100–7.

Robertson MM. The Gilles de la Tourette syndrome: The current status. Arch Dis Child Educ Pract Ed 2012;97:166–75.

Robertson MM. Tourette syndrome, associated conditions and the complexities of treatment. Brain 2000;123:425–62.

Roth J. The colorful spectrum of Tourette syndrome and its medical, surgical and behavioral therapies. Parkinsonism Relat Disord 2018;46(Suppl 1):S75–9.

Serajee FJ, Mahbubul Huq AH. Advances in Tourette syndrome: Diagnoses and treatment. Pediatr Clin North Am 2015;62:687–701.

Shprecher DR, Kious BM, Himle M. Advances in mechanistic understanding and treatment approaches to Tourette syndrome. Discov Med 2015;20:295–301.

Shprecher DR, Schrock L, Himle M. Neurobehavioral aspects, pathophysiology, and management of Tourette syndrome. Curr Opin Neurol 2014;27:484–92.

Singer HS. Motor control, habits, complex motor stereotypies, and Tourette syndrome. Ann N Y Acad Sci 2013;1304:22–31.

Singer HS. Tourette syndrome and other tic disorders. Handb Clin Neurol 2011;100:641–57.

Singer HS. Tourette's syndrome: From behavior to biology. Lancet Neurol 2005;4:149–59.

Stern JS, Burza S, Robertson MM. Gilles de la Tourette's syndrome and its impact in the UK. Postgrad Med J 2005;81:12–19.

Stern JS. Tourette's syndrome and its borderland. Pract Neurol 2018;18:262–70.

Tagwerker Gloor F, Walitza S. Tic disorders and Tourette syndrome: Current concepts of etiology and treatment in children and adolescents. Neuropediatrics 2016;47:84–96.

Thenganatt MA, Jankovic J. Recent advances in understanding and managing Tourette syndrome. F1000Research 2016;5:152.

Trousseau, A. Des diverses espèces de chorées. Clinique Médicale de l'Hôtel Dieu. Paris 1873;2:264–71.

Research Highlights

Black KJ. Tourette syndrome research highlights from 2016. F1000Research 2017;6:1430.

Hartmann A, Worbe Y, Black KJ. Tourette syndrome research highlights from 2017. F1000Research 2018;7:1122.

Mariam N, Cavanna AE. The most cited works in Tourette syndrome. J Child Neurol 2012;27:1250–9.

Richards CA, Black KJ. Tourette syndrome research highlights 2014. F1000Research 2015;4:69.

Richards CA, Black KJ. Tourette syndrome research highlights 2015. F1000Research 2016;5:1493.

Srirathan H, Cavanna AE. Research trends in the neuropsychiatry literature since the new millennium. J Neuropsychiatr Clin Neurosci 2015;27:354–61.

Classification and Epidemiology

Cavanna AE. Improved criteria for the diagnosis of tic disorders in DSM-5. Future Neurol 2014;9:251–3.

Knight T, Steeves T, Day L, Lowerison M, Jette N, Pringsheim T. Prevalence of tic disorders: A systematic review and meta-analysis. Pediatr Neurol 2012;47:77–90.

Robertson MM, Eapen V. Tourette's: syndrome, disorder or spectrum? Classificatory challenges and an appraisal of the DSM criteria. Asian J Psychiatr 2014;11:106–13.

Robertson MM. The prevalence and epidemiology of Gilles de la Tourette syndrome. Part 1: The epidemiological and prevalence studies. J Psychosomatic Res 2008;65:461–72.

Robertson MM. The prevalence and epidemiology of Gilles de la Tourette syndrome. Part 2: Tentative explanations for differing prevalence figures in GTS, including the possible effects of psychopathology, aetiology, cultural differences, and differing phenotypes. J Psychosom Res 2008;65:473–86.

Tourette Syndrome Classification Study Group. Definitions and classification of tic disorders. Arch Neurol 1993;50:1013–16.

Woods DW, Thomsen PH. Tourette and tic disorders in ICD-11: Standing at the diagnostic crossroads. Rev Bras Psiquiatr 2014;36(Suppl 1):51–8.

Premonitory Urges

Belluscio BA, Tinaz S, Hallett M. Similarities and differences between normal urges and the urge to tic. Cogn Neurosci 2011;2:245–6.

Bliss J, Cohen DJ, Freedman DX. Sensory experiences of Gilles de la Tourette syndrome. Arch Gen Psychiatr 1980;37:1343–7.

Cavanna AE, Black KJ, Hallett M, Voon V. Neurobiology of the premonitory urge in Tourette syndrome: Pathophysiology and treatment implications. J Neuropsychiatr Clin Neurosci 2017;29:95–104.

Cavanna AE, Nani A. Tourette syndrome and consciousness of action. Tremor Other Hyperkinetic Mov 2013;3:181.

Conceição VA, Dias Â, Farinha AC, Maia TV. Premonitory urges and tics in Tourette syndrome: Computational mechanisms and neural correlates. Curr Opin Neurobiol 2017;46:187–99.

Cox JH, Seri S, Cavanna AE. Sensory aspects of Tourette syndrome. Neurosci Biobehav Rev 2018;88:170–6.

Ganos C, Hummel FC. My urge, my tic: A missing link between urges and tic inhibition. Cogn Neurosci 2011;2:249–50.

Ganos C, Rothwell J, Haggard P. Voluntary inhibitory motor control over involuntary tic movements. Mov Disord 2018;33:937–46.

Houghton DC, Capriotti MR, Conelea CA, Woods DW. Sensory phenomena in Tourette syndrome: Their role in symptom formation and treatment. Curr Dev Disord Rep 2014;1:245–51.

Jackson GM, Draper A, Dyke K, Pépés SE, Jackson SR. Inhibition, disinhibition and the control of action in Tourette syndrome. Trends Cogn Sci 2015;19:655–65.

Jackson SR, Parkinson A, Kim SY, Schuermann M, Eickhoff SB. On the functional anatomy of the urge-for-action. Cogn Neurosci 2011;2:227–57.

Kane MJ. Premonitory urges as "attentional tics" in Tourette's syndrome. J Am Acad Child Adolesc Psychiatr 1994;33:805–8.

Kranick SM, Hallett M. Neurology of volition. Exp Brain Res 2013;229:313–27.

Patel N, Jankovic J, Hallett M. Sensory aspects of movement disorders. Lancet Neurol 2014;13:100–12.

Prado HS, Rosário MC, Lee J, Hounie AG, Shavitt RG, Miguel EC. Sensory phenomena in obsessive-compulsive disorder and tic disorders: A review of the literature. CNS Spectrums 2008;13:425–32.

Rae CL, Critchley HD, Seth AK. A Bayesian account of the sensory-motor interactions underlying symptoms of Tourette syndrome. Frontiers Psychiatr 2019;10:29.

Behavioural Spectrum

Aldred M, Cavanna AE. Tourette syndrome and socioeconomic status. Neurol Sci 2015;36:1643–9.

Bloch MH, Panza KE, Landeros-Weisenberger A, Leckman JF. Meta-analysis: Treatment of attention-deficit hyperactivity disorder in children with comorbid tic disorders. J Am Acad Child Adolesc Psychiatr 2009;48:884–93.

Cavanna AE, Eddy C, Rickards H. Cognitive functioning in Tourette syndrome. Disc Med 2009;8:191–5.

Cavanna AE, Martino D. How many Gilles de la Tourette syndromes? Eur J Neurol 2014;21:685–6.

Cavanna AE, Servo S, Monaco F, Robertson MM. The behavioral spectrum of Gilles de la Tourette syndrome. J Neuropsychiatr Clin Neurosci 2009;21:13–23.

Cavanna AE. Gilles de la Tourette syndrome as a paradigmatic neuropsychiatric disorder. CNS Spectr 2018;23:213–18.

Cavanna AE. The neuropsychiatry of Gilles de la Tourette syndrome: The état de l'art. Rev Neurol 2018;174:621–7.

Como PG, LaMarsh J, O'Brien KA. Obsessive-compulsive disorder in Tourette's syndrome. Adv Neurol 2005;96:249–61.

Cox JH, Nahar A, Termine C, Agosti M, Balottin U, Seri S, Cavanna AE. Social stigma and self-perception in adolescents with Tourette syndrome. Adolesc Health Med Therapeutics 2019;10:75–82.

Cravedi E, Deniau E, Giannitelli M, Xavier J, Hartmann A, Cohen D. Tourette syndrome and other neurodevelopmental disorders: A comprehensive review. Child Adolesc Psychiatr Ment Health 2017;11:59.

Eapen V, Cavanna AE, Robertson MM. Co-morbidities, social impact and quality of life in Tourette syndrome. Frontiers Psychiatr 2016;7:97.

El Malhany N, Gulisano M, Rizzo R, Curatolo P. Tourette syndrome and comorbid ADHD: Causes and consequences. Eur J Pediatr 2014;174:279–88.

Erenberg G. The relationship between Tourette syndrome, attention deficit hyperactivity disorder, and stimulant medication: A critical review. Semin Pediatr Neurol 2005;12:217–21.

Evans J, Seri S, Cavanna AE. The effects of Gilles de la Tourette syndrome on quality of life across the lifespan: A systematic review. Eur Child Adolesc Psychiatr 2016;25:939–48.

Gagné JP. The psychology of Tourette disorder: Revisiting the past and moving toward a cognitively-oriented future. Clin Psychol Rev 2019;67:11–21.

Kalyva E, Kyriazi M, Vargiami E, Zafeiriou D. A review of co-occurrence of autism spectrum disorder and Tourette syndrome. Res Autism Spectr Disord 2016;24:39–51.

Khalifa N, Von Knorring AL. Psychopathology in a Swedish population of school children with tic disorders. J Am Acad Child Adolesc Psychiatr 2006;45:1346–53.

Kloft L, Steinel T, Kathmann N. Systematic review of co-occurring OCD and TD: Evidence for a tic-related OCD subtype? Neurosci Biobehav Rev 2018;95:280–314.

Lombroso PJ, Scahill L. Tourette syndrome and obsessive-compulsive disorder. Brain Dev 2008;30:231–7.

Martinez-Martin P. What is quality of life and how do we measure it? Relevance to Parkinson's disease and movement disorders. Mov Disord 2017;32:382–92.

Perez DL, Keshavan MS, Scharf JM, Boes AD, Price BH. Bridging the great divide: What can neurology learn from psychiatry? J Neuropsychiatr Clin Neurosci 2018;30:271–8.

Pringsheim T, Piacentini J. Tic-related obsessive-compulsive disorder. J Psychiatr Neurosci 2018;43:431–2.

Rizzo R, Gulisano M, Calì PV, Curatolo P. Tourette syndrome and comorbid ADHD: Current pharmacological treatment options. Eur J Pediatr Neurol 2013;17:421–8.

Robertson MM, Cavanna AE, Eapen V. Gilles de la Tourette syndrome and disruptive behavior disorders: Prevalence, associations and explanation of the relationships. J Neuropsychiatr Clin Neurosci 2015;26:33–41.

Robertson MM. Attention deficit hyperactivity disorder, tics and Tourette's syndrome: The relationship and treatment implications. Eur Child Adolesc Psychiatr 2006;15:1–11.

Robertson MM. Mood disorders and Gilles de la Tourette's syndrome: An update on prevalence, etiology, comorbidity, clinical associations, and implications. J Psychosom Res 2006;61:349–58.

Scahill L, Sukhodolsky DG, Williams SK, Leckman JF. Public health significance of tic disorders and children and adolescents. Adv Neurol 2005;96:240–8.

Silvestri P, Baglioni V, Cardona F, Cavanna AE. Self-concept and self-esteem in patients with chronic tic disorders: A systematic literature review. Eur J Paediatr Neurol 2018;22:749–56.

Simpson HA, Jung L, Murphy TK. Update on attention-deficit/hyperactivity disorder and tic disorders: A review of the current literature. Curr Psychiatr Rep 2011;13:351–6.

Wright A, Rickards H, Cavanna AE. Impulse control disorders in Gilles de la Tourette syndrome. J Neuropsychiatr Clin Neurosci 2012;24:16–27.

Aetiology and Pathophysiology

Albin RL, Mink JW. Recent advances in Tourette syndrome research. Trends Neurosci 2006;29:175–82.

Albin RL. Tourette syndrome: A disorder of the social decision-making network. Brain 2018;141:332–47.

Ali F, Morrison KE, Cavanna AE. The complex genetics of Gilles de la Tourette syndrome: Implications for clinical practice. Neuropsychiatry 2013;3:321–30.

Bronfeld M, Bar-Gad I. Tic disorders: What happens to the basal ganglia? Neuroscientist 2013;19:101–8.

Cauchi RJ, Tarnok Z. Genetic animal models of Tourette syndrome: The long and winding road from lab to clinic. Transl Neurosci 2012;3:153–9.

Cox JH, Seri S, Cavanna AE. Histaminergic modulation in Tourette syndrome. Expert Opinion Orphan Drugs 2016;4:205–13.

Dale RC. Tics and Tourette: A clinical, pathophysiological and etiological review. Curr Opin Pediatr 2017;29:665–73.

Deng H, Gao K, Jankovic J. The genetics of Tourette syndrome. Nat Rev Neurol 2012;8:203–13.

Felling RJ, Singer HS. Neurobiology of Tourette syndrome: Current status and need for further investigation. J Neurosci 2011;31:12387–95.

Ganos C. Tics and Tourette's: Update on pathophysiology and tic control. Curr Opin Neurol 2016;29:513–18.

Hashemiyoon R, Kuhn J, Visser-Vandewalle V. Putting the pieces together in Gilles de la Tourette syndrome: Exploring the link between clinical observations and the biological basis of dysfunction. Brain Topogr 2017;30:3–29.

Hawksley J, Cavanna AE, Nagai Y. The role of the autonomic nervous system in Tourette syndrome. Frontiers Neurosci 2015;9:117.

Leckman JF, Bloch MH, Smith ME, Larabi D, Hampson M. Neurobiological substrates of Tourette's disorder. J Child Adolesc Psychopharmacol 2010;20:237–47.

Madhusudan N, Cavanna AE. The role of immune dysfunction in the development of tics and susceptibility to infections in Tourette syndrome: A systematic review. Basal Ganglia 2013;3:77–84.

Maia TV, Conceição VA. Dopaminergic disturbances in Tourette syndrome: An integrative account. Biol Psychiatr 2018;84:332–44.

Martino D, Ganos C, Worbe Y. Neuroimaging applications in Tourette's syndrome. Int Rev Neurobiol 2018;143:65–108.

Martino D, Zis P, Buttiglione M. The role of immune mechanisms in Tourette syndrome. Brain Res 2015;1617:126–43.

Qi Y, Zheng Y, Li Z, Liu Z, Xiong L. Genetic studies of tic disorders and Tourette syndrome. Methods Mol Biol 2019;2011:547–71.

Zapparoli L, Porta M, Paulesu E. The anarchic brain in action: The contribution of task-based fMRI studies to the understanding of Gilles de la Tourette syndrome. Curr Opin Neurol 2015;28:604–11.

Rating Scales

Cavanna AE, Schrag A, Morley D, Orth M, Robertson MM, Joyce E, Critchley HD, Selai C. The Gilles de la Tourette Syndrome–Quality of Life scale (GTS-QOL): Development and validation. Neurology 2008;71:1410–16.

Chung SJ, Lee JS, Yoo TI, et al. Development of the Korean form of Yale Global Tic Severity Scale: A validity and reliability study. J Korean Neuropsychiatr Assoc 1998;37:942–51.

Cubo E, Saez Velasco S, Delgado Benito V, et al. Validation of screening instruments for neuroepidemiological surveys of tic disorders. Mov Disord 2011;26:520–6.

Gaffney GR, Sieg K, Hellings J. The MOVES: A self-rating scale for Tourette's syndrome. J Child Adolesc Psychopharmacol 1994;4:269–80.

García-López R, Perea-Milla E, Romero-Gonzalez J, et al. Adaptacion al espanol y validez diagnostica de la Yale Global Tics Severity Scale. Rev Neurol 2008;46:261–6.

Gulisano M, Calì P, Palermo F, Robertson MM, Rizzo R. Premonitory urges in patients with Gilles de la Tourette syndrome: An Italian translation and a 7-year follow-up. J Child Adolesc Psychopharmacol 2015;25:810–16.

Jalenques I, Guiguet-Auclair C, Derost P, Joubert P, Foures L, Hartmann A, Muellner J, Rondepierre F. Syndrome de Gilles de La Tourette Study Group. The MOVES (Motor tic, Obsessions and compulsions, Vocal tic Evaluation Survey): Cross-cultural evaluation of the French version and additional psychometric assessment. J Neurol 2018;265:678–87.

Jeon S, Walkup JT, Woods DW, et al. Detecting a clinically meaningful change in tic severity in Tourette syndrome: A comparison of three methods. Contemp Clin Trials 2013;36:414–20.

Kircanski K, Woods DW, Chang SW, Ricketts EJ, Piacentini JC. Cluster analysis of the Yale Global Tic Severity Scale (YGTSS): Symptom dimensions and clinical correlates in an outpatient youth sample. J Abnorm Child Psychol 2010;38:777–88.

Leckman JF, Riddle MA, Hardin MT, et al. The Yale Global Tic Severity Scale: Initial testing of a clinician-rated scale of tic severity. J Am Acad Child Adolesc Psychiatr 1989;28:566–73.

Leckman JF, Towbin KE, Ort SI, Cohen DJ. Clinical assessment of tic disorder severity. In: Cohen DJ, Bruun RD, Leckman JF (eds), Tourette's syndrome and tic disorders: Clinical understanding and treatment. New York: John Wiley, 1988.

Leivonen S, Voutilainen A, Hinkka-Yii-Salomaki S, et al. A nationwide register study of the characteristics, incidence and validity of diagnosed Tourette syndrome and other tic disorders. Acta Paediatr 2014;103:984–90.

Martino D, Cavanna AE, Colosimo C, Hartmann A, Leckman JF, Munchau A, Pringsheim TM. Systematic review of severity scales and screening instruments for tics: Critique and recommendations. Mov Disord 2017;32:467–73.

McGuire JF, McBride N, Piacentini J, et al. The premonitory urge revisited: An individualized premonitory urge for tics scale. J Psychiatr Res 2016;83:176–83.

McGuire JF, Piacentini J, Storch EA, et al. A multicenter examination and strategic revisions of the Yale Global Tic Severity Scale. Neurology 2018;90:e1711–19.

Pietracupa S, Bruno E, Cavanna AE, Falla M, Zappia M, Colosimo C. Scales for hyperkinetic disorders: A systematic review. J Neurol Sci 2015;358:9–21.

Robertson MM, Banerjee S, Kurlan R, Cohen DJ, Leckman JF, McMahon W, Pauls DL, Sandor P, van de Wetering BJ. The Tourette syndrome diagnostic confidence index: Development and clinical associations. Neurology 1999;53:2108–12.

Shapiro AK, Shapiro ES. Controlled study of pimozide vs. placebo in Tourette's syndrome. J Am Acad Child Psychiatr 1984;23:161–73.

Shytle RD, Silver AA, Sheehan KH, et al. The Tourette's Disorder Scale (TODS): Development, reliability, and validity. Assessment 2003;10:273–87.

Stefanoff P, Wolanczyk T. Validity and reliability of Polish adaptation of Yale Global Tic Severity Scale (YGTSS) in a study of Warsaw schoolchildren aged 12–15. Przegl Epidemiol 2005;59:753–62.

Steinberg T, Baruch SS, Harush A, et al. Tic disorders and the premonitory urge. J Neural Transm 2010;117:277–84.

Storch EA, De Nadai AS, Lewin AB, et al. Defining treatment response in pediatric tic disorders: A signal detection analysis of the Yale Global Tic Severity Scale. J Child Adolesc Psychopharmacol 2011;21:621–7.

Storch EA, Merlo LJ, Lehmkuhl H, et al. Further psychometric examination of the Tourette's Disorder Scales. Child Psychiatr Hum Dev 2007;38:89–98.

Storch EA, Murphy TK, Fernandez M, et al. Factor-analytic study of the Yale Global Tic Severity Scale. Psychiatr Res 2007;149:231–7.

Storch EA, Murphy TK, Geffken GR, et al. Further psychometric properties of the Tourette's Disorder Scale-Parent Rated version (TODS-PR). Child Psychiatr Hum Dev 2004;35:107–20.

Storch EA, Murphy TK, Geffken GR, et al. Reliability and validity of the Yale Global Tic Severity Scale. Psychol Assess 2005;17:486–91.

Su MT, McFarlane F, Cavanna AE, Termine C, Murray I, Heidemeyer L, Heyman I, Murphy T. The English version of the Gilles de la Tourette Syndrome–Quality of Life Scale for children and adolescents (C&A-GTS-QOL): A validation study in the United Kingdom. J Child Neurol 2017;32:76–83.

Sutherland Owens AN, Miguel EC, Swerdlow NR. Sensory gating scales and premonitory urges in Tourette syndrome. Sci World J 2011;11:736–41.

Walkup JT, Rosenberg LA, Brown J, Singer HS. The validity of instruments measuring tic severity in Tourette's syndrome. J Am Acad Child Adolesc Psychiatr 1992;31:472–7.

Wang S, Qi F, Li J, Zhao L, Li A. Effects of Chinese herbal medicine Ningdong Granule on regulating dopamine (DA)/serotonin (5-TH) and gamma-aminobutyric acid (GABA) in patients with Tourette syndrome. BioSci Trends 2012;6:212–18.

Woods DW, Piacentini J, Himle MB, Chang S. Premonitory urge for tics scale (PUTS): Initial psychometric results and examination of the premonitory urge phenomenon in youths with tic disorders. Dev Behav Pediatr 2005;26:397–403.

Treatment

Accad M, Francis D. Does evidence based medicine adversely affect clinical judgment? BMJ 2018;362:k2799.

Ackermans L, Kuhn J, Neuner I, Temel Y, Visser-Vandewalle V. Surgery for Tourette syndrome. World Neurosurg 2013;80: e15–22.

Ackermans L, Temel Y, Visser-Vandewalle V. Deep brain stimulation in Tourette's syndrome. Neurotherapeutics 2008;5:339–44.

Akbarian-Tefaghi L, Zrinzo L, Foltynie T. The use of deep brain stimulation in Tourette syndrome. Brain Sci 2016;6:35.

Akici A, Oktay S. Rational pharmacotherapy and pharmacovigilance. Curr Drug Safety 2007;2:65–9.

Baldermann JC, Schüller T, Huys D, Becker I, Timmermann L, Jessen F, Visser-Vandewalle V, Kuhn J. Deep brain stimulation for Tourette syndrome: A systematic review and meta-analysis. Brain Stimul 2016;9:296–304.

Bate KS, Malouff JM, Thorsteinsson ET, Bhullar N. The efficacy of habit reversal therapy for tics, habit disorders, and stuttering: A meta-analytic review. Clin Psychol Rev 2011;31:865–71.

Bennett SM, Keller AE, Walkup JT. The future of tic disorder treatment. Ann N Y Acad Sci 2013;1304:32–9.

Bloch MH. Emerging treatments for Tourette's disorder. Curr Psychiatr Rep 2008;10:323–30.

Budman CL. The role of atypical antipsychotics for treatment of Tourette's syndrome. Drugs 2014;74:1177–93.

Caprini G, Melotti V. Una grave sindrome ticcosa guarita con haloperidol. Rivista Sperimentale di Freniatra 1961;85:191–6.

Cavanna AE, Eddy CM, Mitchell R, Pall H, Mitchell I, Zrinzo L, Foltynie T, Jahanshahi M, Limousin P, Hariz MI, Rickards H. An approach to Deep Brain Stimulation for severe treatment-refractory Tourette syndrome: The UK perspective. Br J Neurosurg 2011;25:38–44.

Cavanna AE, Monaco F. Placebo treatments: Historical overview and current concepts. Confinia Cephalalgica 2006;15:3–11.

Cavanna AE, Nani A. Pharmacological treatment of tics in Gilles de la Tourette syndrome. Clin Manage Issues 2011;5:145–55.

Cavanna AE, Seri S. Chronic tic disorders: Diagnosis, treatment and management. Clinical Pharmacist 2016;8:2.

Cavanna AE, Strigaro G, Monaco F. Brain mechanisms underlying the placebo effect in neurological disorders. Funct Neurol 2007;22:89–94.

Cavanna AE. Back to the future: Stoic wisdom and psychotherapy for neuropsychiatric conditions. Future Neurology 2019;14:1.

Cavanna AE. Stoic philosophy and psychotherapy: Implications for neuropsychiatric conditions. Dialogues Philos Mental Neuro Sci 2019;12:10–24.

Chadehumbe MA, Brown LW. Advances in the treatment of Tourette's disorder. Curr Psychiatr Rep 2019;21:31.

Chandros S, Colloca L, Avins A, Gordon NP, Somkin CP, Kaptchuk TJ, Miller FG. Patients' attitudes about the use of placebo treatments: Telephone survey. BMJ 2013;346:f3757.

Cox JH, Seri S, Cavanna AE. Safety and efficacy of aripiprazole for the treatment of pediatric Tourette syndrome and other chronic tic disorders. Pediatr Health Med Therapeutics 2016;7:57–64.

Cubo E, González M, Singer H, Mahone EM, Scahill L, MüllerVahl KR, et al. Impact of placebo assignment in clinical trials of tic disorders. Mov Disord 2013;28(9):1288–92.

Deeb W, Malaty IA, Mathews CA. Tourette disorder and other tic disorders. Handb Clin Neurol 2019;165:123–53.

Dutta N, Cavanna AE. Effectiveness of Habit Reversal Therapy in the treatment of Tourette syndrome and other chronic tic disorders: A systematic review. Funct Neurol 2013;28:7–12.

Eddy CM, Rickards HE, Cavanna AE. Treatment strategies for tics in Tourette syndrome. Therapeutic Adv Neurol Disord 2011;4:25–45.

Evidence Based Medicine Working Group. Evidence based medicine: A new approach to teaching the practice of medicine. JAMA 1992;268:2420–5.

Faria V, Kossowsky J, Petkov MP, Kaptchuk TJ, Kirsch I, Lebel A, Borsook D. Parental attitudes about placebo use in children. J Pediatr 2017;181:272–8.

Ferreira JJ, Trenkwalder C, Mestre TA. Placebo and nocebo responses in other movement disorders besides Parkinson's disease: How much do we know? Mov Disord 2018;33:1228–35.

Fraint A, Pal G. Deep brain stimulation in Tourette's syndrome. Frontiers Neurol 2015;6:170.

Fründt O, Woods D, Ganos C. Behavioral therapy for Tourette syndrome and chronic tic disorders. Neurol Clin Pract 2017;7:148–56.

Ganos C, Martino D, Pringsheim T. Tics in the pediatric population: Pragmatic management. Mov Disord Clin Pract 2017;4:160–72.

Gordon JA. From neurobiology to novel medications: A principled approach to translation. Am J Psychiatr 2019;176:425–7.

Greenhalgh T, Howick J, Maskrey N, Evidence Based Medicine Renaissance Group. Evidence based medicine: A movement in crisis? BMJ 2014;348:g3725.

Grelotti DJ, Kaptchuk TJ. Placebo by proxy. BMJ 2011;343:d4345.

Hariz MI, Robertson MM. Gilles de la Tourette syndrome and deep brain stimulation. Eur J Neurosci 2010;32:1128–34.

Hartmann A, Martino D, Murphy T. Gilles de la Tourette syndrome: A treatable condition? Rev Neurol 2016;172:446–54.

Huys D, Hardenacke K, Poppe P, Bartch C, Baskin B, Kuhn J. Update on the role of antipsychotics in the treatment of Tourette syndrome. Neuropsychiatric Dis Treatment 2012;8:95–104.

Kermen R, Hickner J, Brody H, Hasham I. Family physicians believe the placebo effect is therapeutic but often use real drugs as placebos. Fam Med 2010;42:636–42.

Kious BM, Jimenez-Shahed J, Shprecher DR. Treatment-refractory Tourette syndrome. Prog Neuropsychopharmacol Biol Psychiatr 2016;70:227–36.

Kompoliti K, Fan W, Leurgans S. Complementary and alternative medicine use in Gilles de la Tourette syndrome. Mov Disord 2009;24:2015–19.

Kompoliti K, Goetz CG, Morrissey M, Leurgans S. Gilles de la Tourette syndrome: Patient's knowledge and concern of adverse effects. Mov Disord 2006;21:248–52.

Koy A, Lin J-P, Sanger TD, Marks WA, Mink JW, Timmermann L. Advances in management of movement disorders in children. Lancet Neurol 2016;15:719–35.

Kurlan RM. Treatment of Tourette syndrome. Neurotherapeutics 2014;11:161–5.

Ludlow AK, Rogers SL. Understanding the impact of diet and nutrition on symptoms of Tourette syndrome: A scoping review. J Child Health Care 2018;22:68–83.

Macerollo A, Martino D, Cavanna AE, Gulisano M, Hartmann A, Hoekstra PJ, Hedderly T, Debes NM, Muller-Vahl K, Neuner I, Porta M, Rickards H, Rizzo R, Cardona F, Roessner V. Refractoriness to pharmacological treatment for tics: A multicenter European audit. J Neurol Sci 2016;366:136–8.

Malaty IA, Akbar U. Updates in medical and surgical therapies for Tourette syndrome. Curr Neurol Neurosci Rep 2014;14:458.

Martino D, Pringsheim TM. Tourette syndrome and other chronic tic disorders: An update on clinical management. Expert Rev Neurother 2018;12:125–37.

McGuire JF, Piacentini J, Brennan EA, Lewin AB, Murphy TK, Small BJ, Storch EA. A meta-analysis of behavior therapy for Tourette Syndrome. J Psychiatr Res 2014;50:106–12.

Mink J, Tourette Syndrome Association. Patient selection and assessment recommendations for deep brain stimulation in Tourette syndrome. Mov Disord 2006;21:1831–8.

Mink J. Clinical review of DBS for Tourette syndrome. Frontiers Biosci 2009;1:72–6.

Naguy A. Clonidine use in psychiatry: Panacea or panache? Pharmacology 2016;98:87–92.

Nussey C, Pistrang N, Murphy T. How does psychoeducation help? A review of the effects of providing information about Tourette syndrome and attention-deficit/hyperactivity disorder. Child Care Health Dev 2013;39:617–27.

Pandey S, Dash D. Progress in pharmacological and surgical management of Tourette syndrome and other chronic tic disorders. Neurologist 2019;24:93–108.

Piacentini J, Woods DW, Scahill L, Wilhelm S, Peterson AL, Chang S, Ginsburg GS, Deckersbach T, Dziura J, Levi-Pearl S, Walkup JT. Behavior therapy for children with Tourette disorder: A randomized controlled trial. JAMA 2010;303:1929–37.

Piedad JCP, Rickards H, Cavanna AE. What patients with Gilles de la Tourette syndrome should be treated with deep brain stimulation and what is the best target? Neurosurgery 2012;71:173–92.

Porta M, Menghetti C, Sassi M, Brambilla A, Defendi S, Servello D, Selvini C, Eddy C, Rickards H, Cavanna AE. Treatment-refractory Tourette syndrome. Ital J Psychopathol 2011;17:225–33.

Quezada J, Coffman KA. Current approaches and new developments in the pharmacological management of Tourette syndrome. CNS Drugs 2018;32:33–45.

Reese HE, Timpano KR, Siev J, Rowley T, Wilhelm S. Behavior therapy for Tourette's syndrome and chronic tic disorder: A web-based video illustration of treatment components. Cogn Behav Pract 2010;17:16–24.

Rickards H, Wood C, Cavanna AE. Hassler and Dieckmann's seminal paper on stereotaxic thalamotomy for Gilles de la Tourette syndrome: Translation and critical reappraisal. Mov Disord 2008;23:1966–72.

Roessner V, Schoenffeld K, Buse J, Bender S, Ehrlich S, Münchau A. Pharmacological treatment of tic disorders and Tourette syndrome. Neuropharmacology 2013;68:143–9.

Sackett DL, Rosenberg WMC, Gray JA, Haynes RB, Richardson WS. Evidence based medicine: What it is and what it isn't. BMJ 1996;312:71–2.

Saleh C, Gonzalez V, Cif L, Coubes P. Deep brain stimulation of the globus pallidus internus and Gilles de la Tourette syndrome: Toward multiple networks modulation. Surg Neurol Int 2012;3(Suppl 2):127–42.

Scahill L, Erenberg G, Berlin CM Jr, Budman C, Coffey BJ, Jankovic J, Kiessling L, King RA, Kurlan R, Lang A, Mink J, Murphy T, Zinner S, Walkup J. Contemporary assessment and pharmacotherapy of Tourette syndrome. NeuroRX 2006;3:192–206.

Scahill L, Woods DW, Himle MB, Peterson AL, Wilhelm S, Piacentini JC, McNaught K, Walkup JT, Mink JW. Current controversies on the role of behavior therapy in Tourette syndrome. Mov Disord 2013;28:1179–83.

Scannell JW, Blanckley A, Boldon H, Warrington B. Diagnosing the decline in pharmaceutical R&D efficiency. Nat Rev Drug Disc 2012;11:191–200.

Schrock LE, Mink JW, Woods DW, Porta M, Servello D, Visser-Vandewalle V, et al. Tourette syndrome deep brain stimulation: A review and updated recommendations. Mov Disord 2015;30:448–71.

Seignot JN. Un cas de Maladie de Tics de Gilles de la Tourette guéri par le R.1625. Ann Médico-Psychologiques 1961;119:578–9.

Shprecher D, Kurlan R. The management of tics. Mov Disord 2009;24:15–24.

Singer HS. Treatment of tics and Tourette syndrome. Curr Treat Options Neurol 2010;12:539–61.

Srour M, Lespérance P, Richer F, Chouinard S. Psychopharmacology of tic disorders. J Can Acad Child Adolesc Psychiatr 2008;17:150–9.

Steeves TD, Fox SH. Neurobiological basis of serotonin-dopamine antagonists in the treatment of Gilles de la Tourette syndrome. Prog Brain Res 2008;172:495–513.

Thomas R, Cavanna AE. The pharmacology of Tourette syndrome. J Neural Transmission 2013;120:689–94.

Viswanathan A, Jimenez-Shahed J, Carvallo JFB, Jankovic J. Deep brain stimulation for Tourette syndrome: Target selection. Stereotact Funct Neurosurg 2012;90:213–24.

Waddington JL. Why does the goalkeeper eschew medication? The challenge of new treatments for Tourette syndrome. Mov Disord 2018;33:1236–7.

Waldon K, Hill S, Termine C, Balottin U, Cavanna AE. Trials of pharmacological interventions for Tourette syndrome: A systematic review. Behav Neurol 2013;26:265–73.

Wieseler B, McGauran N, Kaiser T. New drugs: Where did we go wrong and what can we do better? BMJ 2019;366:l4340.

Wile DJ, Pringsheim TM. Behavior therapy for Tourette syndrome: A systematic review and meta-analysis. Curr Treat Options Neurol 2013;15:385–95.

Wilhelm S, Peterson AL, Piacentini J, Woods DW, Deckersbach T, Sukhodolsky DG, Chang S, Liu H, Dziura J, Walkup JT, Scahill L. Randomized trial of behavior therapy for adults with Tourette syndrome. Arch Gen Psychiatr 2012;69:795–803.

Young SL, Taylor M, Lawrie SM. 'First do no harm': A systematic review of the prevalence and management of antipsychotic adverse effects. J Psychopharmacol 2015;29:353–62.

Guidelines

European Guidelines (2011)

Cath DC, Hedderly T, Ludolph AG, Stern JS, Murphy T, Hartmann A, Czernecki V, Robertson MM, Martino D, Munchau A, Rizzo R, ESSTS Guidelines Group. European clinical guidelines for Tourette syndrome and other tic disorders. Part I: Assessment. Eur Child Adolesc Psychiatr 2011;20:155–71.

Roessner V, Plessen KJ, Rothenberger A, Ludolph AG, Rizzo R, Skov L, Strand G, Stern JS, Termine C, Hoekstra PJ, ESSTS Guidelines Group. European clinical guidelines for Tourette syndrome and other tic disorders. Part II: Pharmacological treatment. Eur Child Adolesc Psychiatr 2011;20:173–96.

Verdellen C, van de Griendt J, Hartmann A, Murphy T, ESSTS Guidelines Group. European clinical guidelines for Tourette syndrome and other tic disorders. Part III: Behavioural and psychosocial interventions.

Eur Child Adolesc Psychiatr
2011;20:197–207.

Muller-Vahl KR, Cath DC, Cavanna AE,
Dehning S, Porta M, Robertson MM, Visser-
Vandewalle V, ESSTS Guidelines Group.
European clinical guidelines for Tourette
syndrome and other tic disorders. Part IV:
Deep brain stimulation. Eur Child Adolesc
Psychiatr 2011;20:209–17.

European Expert Consensus Guidelines (2012)

Cavanna AE, Rickards H, Worrall R,
Hoekstra PJ, Plessen KJ, Roessner V. From
ipse dixit to evidence-based guidelines: On
the optimal management of Tourette
syndrome. Eur J Paediatr Neurol
2012;16:310–11.

Rickards H, Cavanna AE, Worrall R. Treatment
practices in Tourette syndrome: The
European perspective. Eur J Paediatr Neurol
2012;16:361–4.

Canadian Guidelines (2012)

Pringsheim T, Doja A, Gorman D, McKinlay D,
Day L, Billinghurst L, Carroll A, Dion Y,
Luscombe S, Steeves T, Sandor P. Canadian
guidelines for the evidence-based treatment
of tic disorders: Pharmacotherapy. Can
J Psychiatr 2012;57:133–43.

Steeves T, McKinlay D, Gorman D,
Billinghurst L, Day L, Carroll A, Dion Y,
Doja A, Luscombe S, Sandor P,
Pringsheim T. Canadian guidelines for the
evidence-based treatment of tic disorders:
Behavioural therapy, deep brain stimulation
and transcranial magnetic stimulation. Can
J Psychiatr 2012;57:144–51.

US Paediatric Guidelines (2013)

Murphy TK, Lewin AB, Storch EA, Stock S.
Practice parameter for the assessment and
treatment of children and adolescents with
tic disorders. J Am Acad Child Adolescent
Psychiatr 2013;52:1341–59.

UK Paediatric Guidelines (2016)

Cuenca J, Glazebrook C, Kendall T, Hedderly T,
Heyman I, Jackson G, Murphy T, Rickards H,
Robertson M, Stern J, Trayner P, Hollis C.
Perceptions of treatment for tics among
young people with Tourette syndrome and
their parents: A mixed methods study. BMC
Psychiatr 2015;15:46.

Hollis C, Pennant M, Cuenca J, Glazebrook C,
Kendall T, Whittington C, Stockton S,
Larsson L, Bunton P, Dobson S, Groom M,
Hedderly T, Heyman I, Jackson GM,
Jackson S, Murphy T, Rickards H,
Robertson M, Stern J. Clinical effectiveness
and patient perspectives of different
treatment strategies for tics in children and
adolescents with Tourette syndrome:
A systematic review and qualitative analysis.
Health Technol Assess 2016;20(4).

Whittington C, Pennant M, Kendall T,
Glazebrook C, Trayner P, Groom M,
Hedderly T, Heyman I, Jackson G,
Murphy T, Rickards H, Robertson M,
Stern M, Hollis C. Treatments for Tourette
syndrome in children and young people:
A systematic review. J Child Psychol
Psychiatr 2016;57:988–1004.

US Guidelines (2019)

Pringsheim T, Okun MS, Muller-Vahl K,
Martino D, Jankovic J, Cavanna AE,
Woods DW, Robinson M, Jarvie E,
Roessner V, Oskoui M, Holler-Managan Y,
Piacentini J. Practice guideline
recommendations summary: Treatment of tics
in people with Tourette syndrome and chronic
tic disorders. Neurology 2019;92:896–906.

Pringsheim T, Holler-Managan Y, Okun MS,
Jankovic J, Piacentini J, Cavanna AE,
Martino D, Muller-Vahl K, Woods DW,
Robinson M, Jarvie E, Roessner V, Oskoui M.
Comprehensive systematic review summary:
Treatment of tics in people with Tourette
syndrome and chronic tic disorders.
Neurology 2019;92:907–15.

Japanese Expert Consensus Guidelines (2019)

Hamamoto Y, Fujio M, Nonaka M, Matsuda N,
Kono T, Kano Y. Expert consensus on
pharmacotherapy for tic disorders in Japan.
Brain Dev 2019;41:501–6.

Reviews of Guidelines

Yang C, Hao Z, Zhu C, Guo Q, Mu D, Zhang L.
Interventions for tic disorders: An overview
of systematic reviews and meta analyses.
Neurosci Biobehav Rev 2016;63:239–55.

Yang C, Zhang Z, Zhang L, Tian J, Yu D, Wang J,
Yang J. Quality assessment of clinical practice
guidelines on tic disorders with AGREE II
instrument. Psychiatr Res 2018;259:385–91.

Methodology

American Academy of Neurology. Clinical practice guideline process manual, 2011. St. Paul, MN: American Academy of Neurology, 2011.

Guyatt GH, Oxman AD, Vist GE, et al. GRADE: An emerging consensus on rating quality of evidence and strength or recommendations. Br Med J 2008;336:924–6.

Moher D, Liberati A, Tetzlaff J, Altman DG, PRISMA Group. Preferred reporting items for systematic reviews and meta-analyses: The PRISMA statement. PLoS Med 2009;6 (7):e1000097.

Moher D, Schulz KF, Simera I, Altman DG. Guidance for developers of health research reporting guidelines. PLoS Med 2010;7(2): e1000217.

Clinical Neuropsychopharmacology

Elbe D, Black TR, McGrane IR, Procyshyn RM. Clinical handbook of psychotropic drugs for children and adolescents online. 4th ed. Boston, MA: Hogrefe, 2019.

Schatzberg AF, DeBattista C. Schatzberg's manual of clinical psychopharmacology. 9th ed. Washington, DC: American Psychiatric Association Publishing, 2019.

Silberstein SD, Marmura MJ, Yuan H. Essential neuropharmacology: The prescriber's guide. 2nd ed. Cambridge: Cambridge University Press, 2015.

Stahl SM. Stahl's essential psychopharmacology: Prescriber's guide. 6th ed. Cambridge: Cambridge University Press, 2018.

Stahl SM. Stahl's essential psychopharmacology: Prescriber's guide – children and adolescents. Cambridge: Cambridge University Press, 2019.

Taylor DM, Barnes TRE, Young AH. The Maudsley prescribing guidelines in psychiatry. 13th ed. Chichester, UK: Wiley-Blackwell, 2018.

Journal Special Issues

Advances in Neurology 1982;35

Goetz CG, Klawans HL. Gilles de la Tourette on Tourette syndrome. Adv Neurol 1982;35:1–16.

Shapiro AK, Shapiro E. Tourette syndrome: History and present status. Adv Neurol 1982;35:17–23.

Murray TJ. Doctor Samuel Johnson's abnormal movements. Adv Neurol 1982;35:25–30.

Cohen DJ, Detlor J, Shaywitz BA, Leckman JF. Interaction of biological and psychological factors in the natural history of Tourette syndrome: A paradigm for childhood neuropsychiatric disorders. Adv Neurol 1982;35:31–4.

Welch KM. Impairment of cerebral serotonin and energy metabolism during ischemia: Relevance to migraine. Adv Neurol 1982;33:35–40.

Nauta WJ. Limbic innervation of the striatum. Adv Neurol 1982;35:41–7.

Levitt P. Central monoamine neuron systems: Their organization in the developing and mature primate brain and the genetic regulation of their terminal fields. Adv Neurol 1982;35:49–59.

Pickel VM, Joh TH, Reis DJ, Miller RJ. Study of enkephalin-containing neurons and dopaminergic afferents in the neostriatum. Adv Neurol 1982;35:61–7.

Iversen SD, Alpert JE. Functional organization of the dopamine system in normal and abnormal behavior. Adv Neurol 1982;35:69–76.

Bonnet KA. Neurobiological dissection of Tourette syndrome: A neurochemical focus on a human neuroanatomical model. Adv Neurol 1982;35:77–82.

Richardson EP Jr. Neuropathological studies of Tourette syndrome. Adv Neurol 1982;35:83–7.

Sacks OW. Acquired Tourettism in adult life. Adv Neurol 1982;35:89–92.

Jacobs BL, Trulson ME, Heym J, Steinfels GF. On the role of CNS serotonin in the motor abnormalities of Tourette syndrome: Behavioral and single-unit studies. Adv Neurol 1982;35:93–8.

Bunney BS, DeRiemer S. Effect of clonidine on dopaminergic neuron activity in the substantia nigra: Possible indirect mediation by noradrenergic regulation of the serotonergic raphe system. Adv Neurol 1982;35:99–104.

Obeso JA, Rothwell JC, Marsden CD. The neurophysiology of Tourette syndrome. Adv Neurol 1982;35:105–14.

Domino EF, Piggott L, Demetriou S, Culbert J. Visually evoked responses in Tourette syndrome. Adv Neurol 1982;35:115–20.

Buck SH, Yamamura HI. Neuropeptides in normal and pathological basal ganglia. Adv Neurol 1982;35:121–32.

Friedhoff AJ. Receptor maturation in pathogenesis and treatment of Tourette syndrome. Adv Neurol 1982;35:133–40.

Stahl SM, Berger PA. Cholinergic and dopaminergic mechanisms in Tourette syndrome. Adv Neurol 1982;35:141–50.

Javoy-Agid F, Ruberg M, Taquet H, Studler JM, Garbarg M, Llorens C, Schwartz JC, Grouselle D, Lloyd KG, Raisman R, Agid Y. Biochemical neuroanatomy of the human substantia nigra (pars compacta) in normal and Parkinsonian subjects. Adv Neurol 1982;35:151–63.

Walsh FX, Bird ED, Stevens TJ. Monoamine transmitters and their metabolites in the basal ganglia of Huntington's disease and control postmortem brain. Adv Neurol 1982;35:165–9.

Ang L, Borison R, Dysken M, Davis JM. Reduced excretion of MHPG in Tourette syndrome. Adv Neurol 1982;35:171–5.

Singer HS, Tune LE, Butler IJ, Zaczek R, Coyle JT. Clinical symptomatology, CSF neurotransmitter metabolites, and serum haloperidol levels in Tourette syndrome. Adv Neurol 1982;35:177–83.

Koslow SH, Cross CK. Cerebrospinal fluid monoamine metabolites in Tourette syndrome and their neuroendocrine implications. Adv Neurol 1982;35:185–97.

Shaywitz BA, Wolf A, Shaywitz SE, Loomis R, Cohen DJ. Animal models of neuropsychiatric disorders and their relevance for Tourette syndrome. Adv Neurol 1982;35:199–202.

Wolfson L, Brown LL, Makman M, Warner C, Dvorkin B, Katzman R. Dopamine mechanisms in the subthalamic nucleus and possible relationship to hemiballismus and other movement disorders. Adv Neurol 1982;35:203–11.

Weiner WJ, Carvey P, Nausieda PA, Goetz CG, Klawans HL. Effect of chronic levodopa on haloperidol-induced behavioral supersensitivity in the guinea pig. Adv Neurol 1982;35:213–19.

Diamond BI, Reyes MG, Borison R. A new animal model for Tourette syndrome. Adv Neurol 1982;35:221–5.

Essman WB, Essman EJ. Comparative features of an animal model for behavioral and neurochemical change. Adv Neurol 1982;35:227–32.

Knott PJ, Hutson PH. Stress-induced stereotypy in the rat: Neuropharmacological similarities to Tourette syndrome. Adv Neurol 1982;35:233–8.

Ruddle FH. Reverse genetics as a means of understanding and treating genetic disease. Adv Neurol 1982;35:239–42.

Kidd KK, Pauls DL. Genetic hypotheses for Tourette syndrome. Adv Neurol 1982;35:243–9.

Comings DE, Gursey BT, Hecht T, Blume K. HLA typing in Tourette syndrome. Adv Neurol 1982;35:251–3.

Comings DE, Gursey BT, Avelino E, Kopp U, Hanin I. Red blood cell choline in Tourette syndrome. Adv Neurol 1982;35:255–8.

Schoenberg BS. Neuroepidemiologic approach to Tourette syndrome. Adv Neurol 1982;35:259–65.

Lucas AR, Beard CM, Rajput AH, Kurland LT. Tourette syndrome in Rochester, Minnesota, 1968–1979. Adv Neurol 1982;35:267–9.

Kondo K, Nomura Y. Tourette syndrome in Japan: Etiologic considerations based on associated factors and familial clustering. Adv Neurol 1982;35:271–6.

Nomura Y, Segawa M. Tourette syndrome in Oriental children: Clinical and pathophysiological considerations. Adv Neurol 1982;35:277–80.

Mak FL, Chung SY, Lee P, Chen S. Tourette syndrome in the Chinese: A follow-up of 15 cases. Adv Neurol 1982;35:281–3.

Asam U. A follow-up study of Tourette syndrome. Adv Neurol 1982;35:285–6.

Golden GS. Tourette syndrome in children: Ethnic and genetic factors and response to stimulant drugs. Adv Neurol 1982;35:287–9.

Nee LE, Polinsky RJ, Ebert MH. Tourette syndrome: Clinical and family studies. Adv Neurol 1982;35:291–5.

Joschko M, Rourke BP. Neuropsychological dimensions of Tourette syndrome: Test-retest stability and implications for intervention. Adv Neurol 1982;35:297–304.

Incagnoli T, Kane R. Neuropsychological functioning in Tourette syndrome. Adv Neurol 1982;35:305–9.

Sutherland RJ, Kolb B, Schoel WM, Whishaw IQ, Davies D. Neuropsychological assessment of children and adults with Tourette syndrome: A comparison with learning disabilities and schizophrenia. Adv Neurol 1982;35:311–22.

Hagin RA, Beecher R, Pagano G, Kreeger H. Effects of Tourette syndrome on learning. Adv Neurol 1982;35:323–8.

Wilson RS, Garron DC, Tanner CM, Klawans HL. Behavior disturbance in children with Tourette syndrome. Adv Neurol 1982;35:329–33.

Montgomery MA, Clayton PJ, Friedhoff AJ. Psychiatric illness in Tourette syndrome patients and first-degree relatives. Adv Neurol 1982;35:335–9.

Fahn S. The clinical spectrum of motor tics. Adv Neurol 1982;35:341–4.

Goetz CG, Tanner CM, Klawans HL. Compressive neuropathies in Tourette syndrome. Adv Neurol 1982;35:345–7.

Fahn S. A case of post-traumatic tic syndrome. Adv Neurol 1982;35:349–50.

Ludlow CL, Polinsky RJ, Caine ED, Bassich CJ, Ebert MH. Language and speech abnormalities in Tourette syndrome. Adv Neurol 1982;35:351–61.

Nuwer MR. Coprolalia as an organic symptom. Adv Neurol 1982;35:363–8.

van Woert MH, Rosenbaum D, Enna SJ. Overview of pharmacological approaches to therapy for Tourette syndrome. Adv Neurol 1982;35:369–75.

Borison RL, Ang L, Chang S, Dysken M, Comaty JE, Davis JM. New pharmacological approaches in the treatment of Tourette syndrome. Adv Neurol 1982;35:377–82.

Shapiro AK, Shapiro E. Clinical efficacy of haloperidol, pimozide, penfluridol, and clonidine in the treatment of Tourette syndrome. Adv Neurol 1982;35:383–6.

Moldofsky H, Brown GM. Tics and serum prolactin response to pimozide in Tourette syndrome. Adv Neurol 1982;35:387–90.

Leckman JF, Cohen DJ, Detlor J, Young JG, Harcherik D, Shaywitz BA. Clonidine in the treatment of Tourette syndrome: A review of data. Adv Neurol 1982;35:391–401.

Bruun RD. Clonidine treatment of Tourette syndrome. Adv Neurol 1982;35:403–5.

Rosenberg GS, Davis KL. Precursors of acetylcholine: Considerations underlying their use in Tourette syndrome. Adv Neurol 1982;35:407–12.

Shapiro E, Shapiro AK. Tardive dyskinesia and chronic neuroleptic treatment of Tourette patients. Adv Neurol 1982;35:413.

Klawans HL, Nausieda PA, Goetz CC, Tanner CM, Weiner WJ. Tourette-like symptoms following chronic neuroleptic therapy. Adv Neurol 1982;35:415–18.

Fog R, Pakkenberg H, Regeur L, Pakkenberg B. 'Tardive' Tourette syndrome in relation to long-term neuroleptic treatment of multiple tics. Adv Neurol 1982;35:419–21.

Rapoport JL, Nee L, Mitchell S, Polinsky R, Ebert M. Hyperkinetic syndrome and Tourette syndrome. Adv Neurol 1982;35:423–6.

Bogomolny A, Erenberg G, Rothner AD. Behavioral effects of haloperidol in young Tourette syndrome patients. Adv Neurol 1982;35:427–32.

Bruun RD. Dysphoric phenomena associated with haloperidol treatment of Tourette syndrome. Adv Neurol 1982;35:433–6.

Caine ED, Polinsky RJ, Ludlow CL, Ebert MH, Nee LE. Heterogeneity and variability in Tourette syndrome. Adv Neurol 1982;35:437–42.

Advances in Neurology 1992;58

Bruun RD, Budman CL. The natural history of Tourette syndrome. Adv Neurol 1992;58:1–6.

Jankovic J. Diagnosis and classification of tics and Tourette syndrome. Adv Neurol 1992;58:7–14.

Leckman JF, Pauls DL, Peterson BS, Riddle MA, Anderson GM, Cohen DJ. Pathogenesis of Tourette syndrome: Clues from the clinical phenotype and natural history. Adv Neurol 1992;58:15–24.

Lang AE. Clinical phenomenology of tic disorders selected aspects. Adv Neurol 1992;58:25–32.

Cath DC, Hoogduin CA, van de Wetering BJ, van Woerkom TC, Roos RA, Rooymans HG. Tourette syndrome and obsessive-compulsive disorder: An analysis of associated phenomena. Adv Neurol 1992;58:33–41.

Fallon T Jr, Schwab-Stone M. Methodology of epidemiological studies of tic disorders and comorbid psychopathology. Adv Neurol 1992;58:43–53.

Earls F. Psychosocial factors in Tourette syndrome. Adv Neurol 1992;58:55–9.

Apter A, Pauls DL, Bleich A, Zohar AH, Kron S, Ratzoni G, Dycian A, Kotler M, Weizman A, Cohen DJ. A population-based epidemiological study of Tourette syndrome among adolescents in Israel. Adv Neurol 1992;58:61–5.

Kerbeshian J, Burd L. Epidemiology and comorbidity: The North Dakota prevalence studies of Tourette syndrome and other developmental disorders. Adv Neurol 1992;58:67–74.

Kurlan R. Tourette syndrome in a special education population: Hypotheses. Adv Neurol 1992;58:75–81.

Leonard HL, Swedo SE, Rapoport JL, Rickler KC, Topol D, Lee S, Rettew D. Tourette syndrome and obsessive-compulsive disorder. Adv Neurol 1992;58:83–93.

Coffey B, Frazier J, Chen S. Comorbidity, Tourette syndrome, and anxiety disorders. Adv Neurol 1992;58:95–104.

Robertson MM. Self-injurious behavior and Tourette syndrome. Adv Neurol 1992;58:105–14.

Lavoie B, Côté PY, Parent A. Immunohistochemical study of the basal ganglia in normal and parkinsonian monkeys. Adv Neurol 1992;58:115–21.

Anderson GM, Pollak ES, Chatterjee D, Leckman JF, Riddle MA, Cohen DJ. Postmortem analysis of subcortical monoamines and amino acids in Tourette syndrome. Adv Neurol 1992;58:123–33.

Singer HS. Neurochemical analysis of postmortem cortical and striatal brain tissue in patients with Tourette syndrome. Adv Neurol 1992;58:135–44.

Haber SN, Wolfer D. Basal ganglia peptidergic staining in Tourette syndrome: A follow-up study. Adv Neurol 1992;58:145–50.

Pauls DL. Issues in genetic linkage studies of Tourette syndrome: Phenotypic spectrum and genetic model parameters. Adv Neurol 1992;58:151–7.

McMahon WM, Leppert M, Filloux F, van de Wetering BJ, Hasstedt S. Tourette symptoms in 161 related family members. Adv Neurol 1992;58:159–65.

Heutink P, van de Wetering BJ, Breedveld GJ, Oostra BA. Genetic study on Tourette syndrome in the Netherlands. Adv Neurol 1992;58:167–72.

Wilkie PJ, Ahmann PA, Hardacre J, LaPlant RJ, Hiner BC, Weber JL. Application of microsatellite DNA polymorphisms to linkage mapping of Tourette syndrome gene(s). Adv Neurol 1992;58:173–80.

Devor EJ. Linkage studies in 16 St. Louis families: Present status and pursuit of an adjunct strategy. Adv Neurol 1992;58:181–7.

Comings DE, Comings BG. Alternative hypotheses on the inheritance of Tourette syndrome. Adv Neurol 1992;58:189–99.

Demeter S. Structural imaging in Tourette syndrome. Adv Neurol 1992;58:201–6.

Riddle MA, Rasmusson AM, Woods SW, Hoffer PB. SPECT imaging of cerebral blood flow in Tourette syndrome. Adv Neurol 1992;58:207–11.

Stoetter B, Braun AR, Randolph C, Gernert J, Carson RE, Herscovitch P, Chase TN. Functional neuroanatomy of Tourette syndrome: Limbic-motor interactions studied with FDG PET. Adv Neurol 1992;58:213–26.

Brooks DJ, Turjanski N, Sawle GV, Playford ED, Lees AJ. PET studies on the integrity of the pre and postsynaptic dopaminergic system in Tourette syndrome. Adv Neurol 1992;58:227–31.

Singer HS, Wong DF, Brown JE, Brandt J, Krafft L, Shaya E, Dannals RF, Wagner HN Jr. Positron emission tomography evaluation of dopamine D-2 receptors in adults with Tourette syndrome. Adv Neurol 1992;58:233–9.

Erenberg G. Treatment of Tourette syndrome with neuroleptic drugs. Adv Neurol 1992;58:241–3.

Goetz CG. Clonidine and clonazepam in Tourette syndrome. Adv Neurol 1992;58:245–51.

Chappell PB, Leckman JF, Riddle MA, Anderson GM, Listwack SJ, Ort SI, Hardin MT, Scahill LD, Cohen DJ. Neuroendocrine and behavioral effects of naloxone in Tourette syndrome. Adv Neurol 1992;58:253–62.

LeWitt PA. Therapeutics of Tourette syndrome: New medication approaches. Adv Neurol 1992;58:263–70.

Sverd J, Gadow KD, Nolan EE, Sprafkin J, Ezor SN. Methylphenidate in hyperactive boys with comorbid tic disorder. I. Clinic evaluations. Adv Neurol 1992;58:271–81.

King RA, Riddle MA, Goodman WK. Psychopharmacology of obsessive-compulsive disorder in Tourette syndrome. Adv Neurol 1992;58:283–91.

Wurtman RJ. Effects of foods on the brain: Possible implications for understanding and treating Tourette syndrome. Adv Neurol 1992;58:293–301.

Haslam RH. Is there a role for megavitamin therapy in the treatment of attention deficit hyperactivity disorder? Adv Neurol 1992;58:303–10.

Burd L, Kerbeshian J. Educational management of children with Tourette syndrome. Adv Neurol 1992;58:311–17.

Harper G. The family in Tourette syndrome. Adv Neurol 1992;58:319–22.

Nomura Y, Kita M, Segawa M. Social adaptation of Tourette syndrome families in Japan. Adv Neurol 1992;58:323–32.

Baer L. Behavior therapy for obsessive-compulsive disorder and trichotillomania: Implications for Tourette syndrome. Adv Neurol 1992;58:333–40.

Cohen DJ, Friedhoff AJ, Leckman JF, Chase TN. Tourette syndrome: Extending basic research to clinical care. Adv Neurol 1992;58:341–62.

Neurologic Clinics 1997;15

Jankovic J. Preface. Neurol Clin 1997;15:xv–xvi.

Kompoliti K, Goetz CG. Clinical rating and quantitative assessment of tics. Neurol Clin 1997;15:239–54.

Como PG. Neuropsychological tests for obsessive-compulsive disorder and attention deficit hyperactivity disorder. Neurol Clin 1997;15:255–65.

Jankovic J. Phenomenology and classification of tics. Neurol Clin 1997;15:267–75.

Coffey BJ, Park KS. Behavioral and emotional aspects of Tourette syndrome. Neurol Clin 1997;15:277–89.

Bruun RD, Budman CL. The course and prognosis of Tourette syndrome. Neurol Clin 1997;15:291–8.

Singer C. Coprolalia and other coprophenomena. Neurol Clin 1997;15:299–308.

Kumar R, Lang AE. Secondary tic disorders. Neurol Clin 1997;15:309–31.

Hallett JJ, Kiessling SL. Neuroimmunology of tics and other childhood hyperkinesias. Neurol Clin 1997;15:333–44.

Stern JS, Robertson MM. Tics associated with autistic and pervasive developmental disorders. Neurol Clin 1997;15:345–55.

Singer HS. Neurobiology of Tourette syndrome. Neurol Clin 1997;15:357–79.

Alsobrook JP, Pauls DL. The genetics of Tourette syndrome. Neurol Clin 1997;15:381–93.

Tanner CM, Goldman SM. Epidemiology of Tourette syndrome. Neurol Clin 1997;15:395–402.

Kurlan R. Treatment of tics. Neurol Clin 1997;15:403–9.

Freeman RD. Attention deficit hyperactivity disorder in the presence of Tourette syndrome. Neurol Clin 1997;15:411–20.

Rapoport JL, Inoff-Germain G. Medical and surgical treatment of obsessive-compulsive disorder. Neurol Clin 1997;15:421–8.

Chappell PB, Scahill LD, Leckman JF. Future therapies of Tourette syndrome. Neurol Clin 1997;15:429–50.

Kurlan R. Future direction of research in Tourette syndrome. Neurol Clin 1997;15:451–6.

Packer LE. Social and educational resources for patients with Tourette syndrome. Neurol Clin 1997;15:457–73.

CNS Spectrums 1999;4(2)

Hollander E. Clinical aspects of Tourette syndrome. CNS Spectrums 1999;4(2):15–20.

Erenberg G. Toward understanding Tourette syndrome. CNS Spectrums 1999;4(2):21.

Hollenbeck P. How life imitates Tourette syndrome: Reflections of an afflicted neuroscientist. CNS Spectrums 1999;4(2):22–3.

Kushner HI. From Gilles de la Tourette's disease to Tourette syndrome: A history. CNS Spectrums 1999;4(2):24–35.

Erenberg G. The clinical neurology of Tourette syndrome. CNS Spectrums 1999;4(2):36–53.

Walkup JT. The psychiatry of Tourette syndrome. CNS Spectrums 1999;4(2):54–61.

Kurlan R. Investigating Tourette syndrome as a neurologic sequela of rheumatic fever. CNS Spectrums 1999;4(2):62–7.

Silver AA, Douglas Shytle R, Sanberg PR. Clinical experience with transdermal nicotine patch in Tourette syndrome. CNS Spectrums 1999;4(2):68–76.

Guarda AS, Treasure J, Robertson MM. Eating disorders and Tourette syndrome: A case series of comorbidity and associated obsessive-compulsive symptomatology. CNS Spectrums 1999;4(2):77–80.

CNS Spectrums 1999;4(3)

Hollander E. The neuroscience of the Tourette syndrome spectrum. CNS Spectrums 1999;4 (3):13–15.

Swerdlow NR. Tourette syndrome: Lessons from a model. CNS Spectrums 1999;4 (3):16–17.

Fuerst ML. An interview with Jim Eisenreich. CNS Spectrums 1999;4(3):18–20.

Swerdlow NR, Zinner S, Farber RH, Seacrist C, Hartston H. Symptoms in obsessive-compulsive disorder and Tourette syndrome: A spectrum? CNS Spectrums 1999;4(3):21–33.

Alsobrook JP. The genetics of Tourette syndrome. CNS Spectrums 1999;4(3):34–53.

Wright CI, Peterson BS, Rauch SL. Neuroimaging studies in Tourette syndrome. CNS Spectrums 1999;4(3):54–61.

Swerdlow NR, Young AB. Neuropathology in Tourette syndrome. CNS Spectrums 1999;4 (3):65–74.

Advances in Neurology 2001;85

Leckman JF, Peterson BS, King RA, Scahill L, Cohen DJ. Phenomenology of tics and natural history of tic disorders. Adv Neurol 2001;85:1–14.

Jankovic J. Differential diagnosis and etiology of tics. Adv Neurol 2001;85:15–29.

Goetz CG, Kompoliti K. Rating scales and quantitative assessment of tics. Adv Neurol 2001;85:31–42.

Miguel EC, do Rosário-Campos MC, Shavitt RG, Hounie AG, Mercadante MT. The tic-related obsessive-compulsive disorder phenotype and treatment implications. Adv Neurol 2001;85:43–55.

Spencer T, Biederman J, Coffey B, Geller D, Faraone S, Wilens T. Tourette disorder and ADHD. Adv Neurol 2001;85:57–77.

King RA, Scahill L. Emotional and behavioral difficulties associated with Tourette syndrome. Adv Neurol 2001;85:79–88.

Rapin I. Autism spectrum disorders: Relevance to Tourette syndrome. Adv Neurol 2001;85:89–101.

Como PG. Neuropsychological function in Tourette syndrome. Adv Neurol 2001;85:103–11.

Mink JW. Neurobiology of basal ganglia circuits in Tourette syndrome: Faulty inhibition of unwanted motor patterns? Adv Neurol 2001;85:113–22.

Graybiel AM, Canales JJ. The neurobiology of repetitive behaviors: Clues to the neurobiology of Tourette syndrome. Adv Neurol 2001;85:123–31.

Walters JR, Ruskin DN, Baek D, Allers KA, Bergstrom DA. Cognitive function paradigms: Implications of neurophysiological studies of dopamine stimulants for Tourette syndrome and comorbid attention-deficit hyperactivity disorder. Adv Neurol 2001;85:133–49.

Swerdlow NR, Young AB. Neuropathology in Tourette syndrome: An update. Adv Neurol 2001;85:151–61.

Singer HS, Wendlandt JT. Neurochemistry and synaptic neurotransmission in Tourette syndrome. Adv Neurol 2001;85:163–78.

Peterson BS. Neuroimaging studies of Tourette syndrome: A decade of progress. Adv Neurol 2001;85:179–96.

Castellanos FX. Neural substrates of attention-deficit hyperactivity disorder. Adv Neurol 2001;85:197–206.

Rauch SL, Whalen PJ, Curran T, Shin LM, Coffey BJ, Savage CR, McInerney SC, Baer L, Jenike MA. Probing striato-thalamic function in obsessive-compulsive disorder and Tourette syndrome using neuroimaging methods. Adv Neurol 2001;85:207–24.

George MS, Sallee FR, Nahas Z, Oliver NC, Wassermann EM. Transcranial magnetic stimulation (TMS) as a research tool in Tourette syndrome and related disorders. Adv Neurol 2001;85:225–35.

Hallett M. Neurophysiology of tics. Adv Neurol 2001;85:237–44.

Rothenberger A, Kostanecka T, Kinkelbur J, Cohrs S, Woerner W, Hajak G. Sleep and Tourette syndrome. Adv Neurol 2001;85:245–59.

Scahill L, Tanner C, Dure L. The epidemiology of tics and Tourette syndrome in children and adolescents. Adv Neurol 2001;85:261–71.

Walkup JT. Epigenetic and environmental risk factors in Tourette syndrome. Adv Neurol 2001;85:273–9.

Pauls DL, Tourette Syndrome Association International Consortium on Genetics. Update on the genetics of Tourette syndrome. Adv Neurol 2001;85:281–93.

Bessen DE, Lombroso PJ. Group A streptococcal infections and their potential role in neuropsychiatric disease. Adv Neurol 2001;85:295–305.

Kurlan R. Could Tourette syndrome be a neurologic manifestation of rheumatic fever? Adv Neurol 2001;85:307–10.

Hamilton CS, Garvey MA, Swedo SE. Therapeutic implications of immunology for tics and obsessive-compulsive disorder. Adv Neurol 2001;85:311–18.

Piacentini J, Chang S. Behavioral treatments for Tourette syndrome and tic disorders: State of the art. Adv Neurol 2001;85:319–31.

Arnsten AF. Modulation of prefrontal cortical-striatal circuits: Relevance to therapeutic treatments for Tourette syndrome and attention-deficit hyperactivity disorder. Adv Neurol 2001;85:333–41.

Riddle MA, Carlson J. Clinical psychopharmacology for Tourette syndrome and associated disorders. Adv Neurol 2001;85:343–54.

Lang AE. Update on the treatment of tics. Adv Neurol 2001;85:355–62.

Hollenbeck PJ. Insight and hindsight into Tourette syndrome. Adv Neurol 2001;85:363–7.

Leckman JF, Cohen DJ, Goetz CG, Jankovic J. Tourette syndrome: Pieces of the puzzle. Adv Neurol 2001;85:369–90.

Brain and Development 2003;25(Suppl. 1)

Segawa M, Nomura Y. Preface. Brain Develop 2003;25(Suppl. 1):S1–2.

Groenewegen HJ, van den Heuvel OA, Cath DC, Voorn P, Veltman DJ. Does an imbalance between the dorsal and ventral striatopallidal systems play a role in Tourette's syndrome? A neuronal circuit approach. Brain Develop 2003;25(Suppl. 1):S3–14.

Saka E, Graybiel AM. Pathophysiology of Tourette's syndrome: Striatal pathways revisited. Brain Develop 2003;25(Suppl. 1): S15–19.

Kimura M, Yamada H, Matsumoto N. Tonically active neurons in the striatum encode motivational contexts of action. Brain Develop 2003;25(Suppl. 1):S20–3.

Leckman JF. Phenomenology of tics and natural history of tic disorders. Brain Develop 2003;25(Suppl. 1):S24–8.

Wang H-S, Kuo M-F. Tourette's syndrome in Taiwan: An epidemiological study of tic disorders in an elementary school at Taipei County. Brain Develop 2003;25(Suppl. 1): S29–31.

Ohta M, Kano Y. Clinical characteristics of adult patients with tics and/or Tourette's syndrome. Brain Develop 2003;25(Suppl. 1): S32–6.

Nomura Y, Segawa M. Neurology of Tourette's syndrome (TS) – TS as a developmental dopamine disorder: A hypothesis. Brain Develop 2003;25(Suppl. 1):S37–42.

Wang H-S, Kuo M-F. Sonographic lenticulostriate vasculopathy in infancy with tic and other neuropsychiatric disorders developed after 7 to 9 years of follow-up. Brain Develop 2003;25(Suppl. 1):S43–7.

Nomura Y, Fukuda H, Terao Y, Hikosaka O, Segawa M. Abnormalities of voluntary saccades in Gilles de la Tourette's syndrome: Pathophysiological consideration. Brain Develop 2003;25(Suppl. 1):S48–54.

Grados MA, Walkup J, Walford S. Genetics of obsessive-compulsive disorders: New findings and challenges. Brain Develop 2003;25(Suppl. 1):S55–61.

Segawa M. Neurophysiology of Tourette's syndrome: Pathophysiological considerations. Brain Develop 2003;25 (Suppl. 1):S62–9.

Singer HS, Minzer K. Neurobiology of Tourette's syndrome: Concepts of neuroanatomic localization and neurochemical abnormalities. Brain Develop 2003;25(Suppl. 1):S70–84.

Journal of Psychosomatic Research 2003;55(1)

Sandor P. From the editor. J Psychosom Res 2003;55(1):1–2.

Robertson MM. Diagnosing Tourette syndrome: Is it a common disorder? J Psychosom Res 2003;55(1):3–6.

Pauls DL. An update on the genetics of Gilles de la Tourette syndrome. J Psychosom Res 2003;55(1):7–12.

Gerard E, Peterson BS. Developmental processes and brain imaging studies in Tourette syndrome. J Psychosom Res 2003;55 (1):13–22.

Kostanecka-Endress T, Banaschewski T, Kinkelbur J, Wüllner I, Lichtblau S, Cohrs S, Rüther E, Woerner W, Hajak G, Rothenberger A. Disturbed sleep in children with Tourette syndrome: A polysomnographic study. J Psychosom Res 2003;55(1):23–9.

Singer HS, Loiselle C. PANDAS: A commentary. J Psychosom Res 2003;55(1):31–9.

Sandor P. Pharmacological management of tics in patients with TS. J Psychosom Res 2003;55 (1):41–8.

Miguel EC, Shavitt RG, Ferrão YA, Brotto SA, Diniz JB. How to treat OCD in patients with Tourette syndrome. J Psychosom Res 2003;55 (1):49–57.

Budman CL, Rockmore L, Stokes J, Sossin M. Clinical phenomenology of episodic rage in children with Tourette syndrome. J Psychosom Res 2003;55(1):59–65.

Greene RW, Ablon JS, Goring JC. A transactional model of oppositional behavior: Underpinnings of the collaborative problem solving approach. J Psychosom Res 2003;55(1):67–75.

Behavior Modification 2005;29(5–6)

Woods DW. Introduction to the special issue on the Clinical Management of Tourette's Syndrome: A behavioral perspective. Behav Modification 2005;29(5–6):711–15.

Meidinger AL, Miltenberger RG, Himle M, Omvig M, Trainor C, Crosby R. An investigation of tic suppression and the rebound effect in Tourette's disorder. Behav Modification 2005;29(5–6):716–45.

Osmon DC, Smerz JM. Neuropsychological evaluation in the diagnosis and treatment of Tourette's syndrome. Behav Modification 2005;29(5–6):746–83.

Mansueto CS, Keuler DJ. Tic or compulsion? It's Tourettic OCD. Behav Modification 2005;29 (5–6):784–99.

Piacentini J, Chang S. Habit reversal training for tic disorders in children and adolescents. Behav Modification 2005;29(5–6):803–22.

Gilman R, Connor N, Haney M. A school-based application of modified habit reversal for Tourette syndrome via a translator: A case study. Behav Modification 2005;29 (5–6):823–38.

Watson TS, Dufrene B, Weaver A, Butler T, Meeks C. Brief antecedent assessment and treatment of tics in the general education classroom: A preliminary investigation. Behav Modification 2005;29(5–6):839–57.

Carr JE, Chong IM. Habit reversal treatment of tic disorders: A methodological critique of the literature. Behav Modification 2005;29 (5–6):858–75.

Packer LE. Tic-related school problems: Impact on functioning, accommodations, and interventions. Behav Modification 2005;29 (5–6):876–99.

Woods DW, Marcks BA. Controlled evaluation of an educational intervention used to modify peer attitudes and behavior toward persons with Tourette's syndrome. Behav Modification 2005;29(5–6):900–12.

Advances in Neurology 2006;99

Leckman JF, Bloch MH, King RA, Scahill L. Phenomenology of tics and natural history of tic disorders. Adv Neurol 2006;99:1–16.

Denckla MB. Attention deficit hyperactivity disorder: The childhood co-morbidity that most influences the disability burden in Tourette syndrome. Adv Neurol 2006;99:17–21.

Hounie AG, do Rosario-Campos MC, Diniz JB, Shavitt RG, Ferrão YA, Lopes AC, Mercadante MT, Busatto GF, Miguel EC. Obsessive-compulsive disorder in Tourette syndrome. Adv Neurol 2006;99:22–38.

Robertson MM, Orth M. Behavioral and affective disorders in Tourette syndrome. Adv Neurol 2006;99:39–60.

Jankovic J, Mejia NI. Tics associated with other disorders. Adv Neurol 2006;99:61–8.

Swerdlow NR, Sutherland AN. Preclinical models relevant to Tourette syndrome. Adv Neurol 2006;99:69–88.

Mink JW. Neurobiology of basal ganglia and Tourette syndrome: Basal ganglia circuits and thalamocortical outputs. Adv Neurol 2006;99:89–98.

Albin RL. Neurobiology of basal ganglia and Tourette syndrome: Striatal and dopamine function. Adv Neurol 2006;99:99–106.

Gilbert DL. Motor cortex inhibitory function in Tourette syndrome, attention deficit disorder, and obsessive compulsive disorder:

Studies using transcranial magnetic stimulation. Adv Neurol 2006;99:107–14.

Butler T, Stern E, Silbersweig D. Functional neuroimaging of Tourette syndrome: Advances and future directions. Adv Neurol 2006;99:115–29.

Pauls DL. A genome-wide scan and fine mapping in Tourette syndrome families. Adv Neurol 2006;99:130–5.

McMahon WM, Illmann CL, McGinn MM. Web-based consensus diagnosis for genetics studies of Gilles de la Tourette syndrome. Adv Neurol 2006;99:136–43.

King NM. Genes and Tourette syndrome: Scientific, ethical, and social implications. Adv Neurol 2006;99:144–7.

Murphy TK, Husted DS, Edge PJ. Preclinical/clinical evidence of central nervous system infectious etiology in PANDAS. Adv Neurol 2006;99:148–58.

Giovannoni G. PANDAS: Overview of the hypothesis. Adv Neurol 2006;99:159–65.

Singer HS, Williams PN. Autoimmunity and pediatric movement disorders. Adv Neurol 2006;99:166–78.

King RA. PANDAS: To treat or not to treat? Adv Neurol 2006;99:179–83.

Scahill L, Williams S, Schwab-Stone M, Applegate J, Leckman JF. Disruptive behavior problems in a community sample of children with tic disorders. Adv Neurol 2006;99:184–90.

Dure LS 4th, DeWolfe J. Treatment of tics. Adv Neurol 2006;99:191–6.

Gadow KD, Sverd J. Attention deficit hyperactivity disorder, chronic tic disorder, and methylphenidate. Adv Neurol 2006;99:197–207.

Coffey BJ, Shechter RL. Treatment of co-morbid obsessive compulsive disorder, mood, and anxiety disorders. Adv Neurol 2006;99:208–21.

Budman CL. Treatment of aggression in Tourette syndrome. Adv Neurol 2006;99:222–6.

Piacentini JC, Chang SW. Behavioral treatments for tic suppression: Habit reversal training. Adv Neurol 2006;99:227–33.

Woods DW, Himle MB, Conelea CA. Behavior therapy: Other interventions for tic disorders. Adv Neurol 2006;99:234–40.

Malone DA Jr, Pandya MM. Behavioral neurosurgery. Adv Neurol 2006;99:241–7.

Kurlan R. Future and alternative therapies in Tourette syndrome. Adv Neurol 2006;99:248–53.

Journal of Child Neurology 2006;21(8)

Maria BL. Neurobiology of disease in children: Tourette syndrome. J Child Neurol 2006;21(8):627–8.

Mink JW, Hollenbeck PJ, Swerdlow NR, Levi-Pearl S. Tourette syndrome research. J Child Neurol 2006;21(8):629.

Olson LL, Singer HS, Goodman WK, Maria BL. Tourette syndrome: Diagnosis, strategies, therapies, pathogenesis, and future research directions. J Child Neurol 2006;21(8):630–41.

Leckman JF, Bloch MH, Scahill L, King RA. Tourette syndrome: The self under siege. J Child Neurol 2006;21(8):642–9.

Scahill L, Sukhodolsky DG, Bearss K, Findley D, Hamrin V, Carroll DH, Rains AL. Randomized trial of parent management training in children with tic disorders and disruptive behavior. J Child Neurol 2006;21(8):650–6.

Gaze C, Kepley HO, Walkup JT. Co-occurring psychiatric disorders in children and adolescents with Tourette syndrome. J Child Neurol 2006;21(8):657–64.

Keen-Kim D, Freimer NB. Genetics and epidemiology of Tourette syndrome. J Child Neurol 2006;21(8):665–71.

Frey KA, Albin RL. Neuroimaging of Tourette syndrome. J Child Neurol 2006;21(8):672–7.

Harris K, Singer HS. Tic disorders: Neural circuits, neurochemistry, and neuroimmunology. J Child Neurol 2006;21(8):678–89.

Gilbert D. Treatment of children and adolescents with tics and Tourette syndrome. J Child Neurol 2006;21(8):690–700.

Denckla MB. Attention-deficit hyperactivity disorder (ADHD) comorbidity: A case for "pure" Tourette syndrome? J Child Neurol 2006;21(8):701–3.

Goodman WK, Storch EA, Geffken GR, Murphy TK. Obsessive-compulsive disorder in Tourette syndrome. J Child Neurol 2006;21(8):704–14.

Neimat JS, Patil PG, Lozano AM. Novel surgical therapies for Tourette syndrome. J Child Neurol 2006;21(8):715–18.

Himle MB, Woods DW, Piacentini JC, Walkup JT. Brief review of habit reversal training for Tourette syndrome. J Child Neurol 2006;21(8):719–25.

European Child and Adolescent Psychiatry 2007;16(Suppl. 1)

Rothenberger A, Roessner V, Banaschewski T, Leckman JF. Co-existence of tic disorders and attention-deficit/hyperactivity disorder – recent advances in understanding and treatment. Eur Child Adolesc Psychiatr 2007;16(Suppl. 1):S1–4.

Banaschewski T, Neale BM, Rothenberger A, Roessner V. Comorbidity of tic disorders and ADHD: Conceptual and methodological considerations. Eur Child Adolesc Psychiatr 2007;16(Suppl. 1):S5–14.

Freeman RD, Tourette Syndrome International Database Consortium. Tic disorders and ADHD: Answers from a world-wide clinical dataset on Tourette syndrome. Eur Child Adolesc Psychiatr 2007;16(Suppl. 1):S15–23.

Roessner V, Becker A, Banaschewski T, Freeman RD, Rothenberger A, Tourette Syndrome International Database Consortium. Developmental psychopathology of children and adolescents with Tourette syndrome: Impact of ADHD. Eur Child Adolesc Psychiatr 2007;16(Suppl. 1):S24–35.

Roessner V, Becker A, Banaschewski T, Rothenberger A. Executive functions in children with chronic tic disorders with/ without ADHD: New insights. Eur Child Adolesc Psychiatr 2007;16(Suppl. 1):S36–44.

Kirov R, Banaschewski T, Uebel H, Kinkelbur J, Rothenberger A. REM-sleep alterations in children with co-existence of tic disorders and attention-deficit/hyperactivity disorder: Impact of hypermotor symptoms. Eur Child Adolesc Psychiatr 2007;16(Suppl. 1):S45–50.

Sukhodolsky DG, Leckman JF, Rothenberger A, Scahill L. The role of abnormal neural oscillations in the pathophysiology of co-occurring Tourette syndrome and attention-deficit/hyperactivity disorder. Eur Child Adolesc Psychiatr 2007;16(Suppl. 1):S51–9.

Plessen KJ, Royal JM, Peterson BS. Neuroimaging of tic disorders with co-existing attention-deficit/hyperactivity disorder. Eur Child Adolesc Psychiatr 2007;16(Suppl. 1):S60–70.

Hoekstra PJ, Anderson GM, Troost PW, Kallenberg CG, Minderaa RB. Plasma kynurenine and related measures in tic disorder patients. Eur Child Adolesc Psychiatr 2007;16(Suppl. 1):S71–7.

Poncin Y, Sukhodolsky DG, McGuire J, Scahill L. Drug and non-drug treatments of children with ADHD and tic disorders. Eur Child Adolesc Psychiatr 2007;16(Suppl. 1): S78–88.

Döpfner M, Rothenberger A. Behavior therapy in tic-disorders with co-existing ADHD. Eur Child Adolesc Psychiatr 2007;16(Suppl. 1): S89–99.

Journal of Psychosomatic Research 2009;67(6)

Robertson MM, Cavanna AE. The many faces of Gilles de la Tourette syndrome. J Psychosom Res 2009;67(6):467–8.

Rickards H, Cavanna AE. Gilles de la Tourette: The man behind the syndrome. J Psychosom Res 2009;67(6):469–74.

Robertson MM, Eapen V, Cavanna AE. The international prevalence, epidemiology and clinical phenomenology of Tourette syndrome: A cross-cultural perspective. J Psychosom Res 2009;67(6):475–83.

Monaco F, Servo S, Cavanna AE. Famous people with Gilles de la Tourette syndrome? J Psychosom Res 2009;67(6):485–90.

Grados MA, Mathews CA. Clinical phenomenology and phenotype variability in Tourette syndrome. J Psychosom Res 2009;67(6):491–6.

Bloch MH, Leckman JF. Clinical course of Tourette syndrome. J Psychosom Res 2009;67(6):497–501.

Eddy CM, Rizzo R, Cavanna AE. Neuropsychological aspects of Tourette syndrome: A review. J Psychosom Res 2009;67(6):503–13.

Kerbeshian J, Peng CZ, Burd L. Tourette syndrome and comorbid early-onset schizophrenia. J Psychosom Res 2009;67(6):515–23.

Eapen V, Crncec R. Tourette syndrome in children and adolescents: Special considerations. J Psychosom Res 2009;67(6):525–32.

O'Rourke JA, Scharf JM, Yu D, Pauls DL. The genetics of Tourette syndrome: A review. J Psychosom Res 2009;67(6):533–45.

Martino D, Defazio G, Giovannoni G. The PANDAS subgroup of tic disorders and childhood-onset obsessive-compulsive disorder. J Psychosom Res 2009;67 (6):547–57.

Plessen KJ, Bansal R, Peterson BS. Imaging evidence for anatomical disturbances and neuroplastic compensation in persons with Tourette syndrome. J Psychosom Res 2009;67 (6):559–73.

Rickards H. Functional neuroimaging in Tourette syndrome. J Psychosom Res 2009;67 (6):575–84.

Porta M, Sassi M, Ali F, Cavanna AE, Servello D. Neurosurgical treatment for Gilles de la Tourette syndrome: The Italian perspective. J Psychosom Res 2009;67(6):585–90.

Orth M. Transcranial magnetic stimulation in Gilles de la Tourette syndrome. J Psychosom Res 2009;67(6):591–8.

Nagai Y, Cavanna AE, Critchley HD. Influence of sympathetic arousal on tics: Implications for a therapeutic behavioral intervention for Tourette syndrome. J Psychosom Res 2009;67 (6):599–605.

Journal of Child and Adolescent Psychopharmacology 2010;20(4)

Coffey BJ, Rapoport J. Obsessive-compulsive disorder and Tourette's disorder: Where are we now? J Child Adolesc Psychopharmacol 2010;20(4):235–6.

Leckman JF, Bloch MH, Smith ME, Larabi D, Hampson M. Neurobiological substrates of Tourette's disorder. J Child Adolesc Psychopharmacol 2010;20(4):237–47.

Párraga HC, Harris KM, Párraga KL, Balen GM, Cruz C. An overview of the treatment of Tourette's disorder and tics. J Child Adolesc Psychopharmacol 2010;20(4):249–62.

Wu SW, Harris E, Gilbert DL. Tic suppression: The medical model. J Child Adolesc Psychopharmacol 2010;20(4):263–76.

Kompoliti K, Stebbins GT, Goetz CG, Fan W. Association between antipsychotics and body mass index when treating patients with tics. J Child Adolesc Psychopharmacol 2010;20 (4):277–81.

Lyon GJ, Samar SM, Conelea C, Trujillo MR, Lipinski CM, Bauer CC, Brandt BC, Kemp JJ, Lawrence ZE, Howard J, Castellanos FX, Woods D, Coffey BJ. Testing tic suppression: Comparing the effects of

dexmethylphenidate to no medication in children and adolescents with attention-deficit/hyperactivity disorder and Tourette's disorder. J Child Adolesc Psychopharmacol 2010;20(4):283–9.

Cui YH, Zheng Y, Yang YP, Liu J, Li J. Effectiveness and tolerability of aripiprazole in children and adolescents with Tourette's disorder: A pilot study in China. J Child Adolesc Psychopharmacol 2010;20(4):291–8.

Mancuso E, Faro A, Joshi G, Geller DA. Treatment of pediatric obsessive-compulsive disorder: A review. J Child Adolesc Psychopharmacol 2010;20 (4):299–308.

Grant P, Song JY, Swedo SE. Review of the use of the glutamate antagonist riluzole in psychiatric disorders and a description of recent use in childhood obsessive-compulsive disorder. J Child Adolesc Psychopharmacol 2010;20 (4):309–15.

Murphy TK, Kurlan R, Leckman J. The immunobiology of Tourette's disorder, pediatric autoimmune neuropsychiatric disorders associated with Streptococcus, and related disorders: A way forward. J Child Adolesc Psychopharmacol 2010;20 (4):317–31.

Bernstein GA, Victor AM, Pipal AJ, Williams KA. Comparison of clinical characteristics of pediatric autoimmune neuropsychiatric disorders associated with streptococcal infections and childhood obsessive-compulsive disorder. J Child Adolesc Psychopharmacol 2010;20 (4):333–40.

Behavioural Neurology 2013;27(1)

Cavanna AE. Researching Tourette syndrome in Europe. Behav Neurol 2013;27(1):1–2.

Rickards H, Paschou P, Rizzo R, Stern JS. A brief history of the European Society for the Study of Tourette Syndrome. Behav Neurol 2013;27(1):3–5.

Mol Debes NM. Co-morbid disorders in Tourette syndrome. Behav Neurol 2013;27 (1):7–14.

Eddy CM, Cavanna AE. Altered social cognition in Tourette syndrome: Nature and implications. Behav Neurol 2013;27 (1):15–22.

Elamin I, Edwards MJ, Martino D. Immune dysfunction in Tourette syndrome. Behav Neurol 2013;27(1):23–32.

Eichele H, Plessen KJ. Neural plasticity in functional and anatomical MRI studies of children with Tourette syndrome. Behav Neurol 2013;27(1):33–45.

Rothenberger A, Roessner V. Functional neuroimaging investigations of motor networks in Tourette syndrome. Behav Neurol 2013;27(1):47–55.

Orth M, Münchau A. Transcranial magnetic stimulation studies of sensorimotor networks in Tourette syndrome. Behav Neurol 2013;27(1):57–64.

Rajagopal S, Seri S, Cavanna AE. Premonitory urges and sensorimotor processing in Tourette syndrome. Behav Neurol 2013;27(1):65–73.

Beetsma DJ, van den Hout MA, Engelhard IM, Rijkeboer MM, Cath DC. Does repeated ticking maintain tic behavior? An experimental study of eye blinking in healthy individuals. Behav Neurol 2013;27(1):75–82.

Cavanna AE, David K, Bandera V, Termine C, Balottin U, Schrag A, Selai C. Health-related quality of life in Gilles de la Tourette syndrome: A decade of research. Behav Neurol 2013;27(1):83–93.

Cavanna AE, Luoni C, Selvini C, Blangiardo R, Eddy CM, Silvestri P, Calì P, Seri S, Balottin U, Cardona F, Rizzo R, Termine C. The Gilles de la Tourette Syndrome-Quality of Life Scale for Children and Adolescents (GTS-QOL-C&A): Development and validation of the Italian version. Behav Neurol 2013;27(1):95–103.

Frank M, Cavanna AE. Behavioural treatments for Tourette syndrome: An evidence-based review. Behav Neurol 2013;27(1):105–17.

Müller-Vahl KR. Treatment of Tourette syndrome with cannabinoids. Behav Neurol 2013;27(1):119–24.

Porta M, Cavanna AE, Zekaj E, D'Adda F, Servello D. Selection of patients with Tourette syndrome for Deep Brain Stimulation (DBS) surgery. Behav Neurol 2013;27(1):125–31.

Ackermans L, Neuner I, Temel Y, Duits A, Kuhn J, Visser-Vandewalle V. Thalamic deep brain stimulation for Tourette syndrome. Behav Neurol 2013;27(1):133–8.

Cavanna AE, Kavanagh C, Robertson MM. The future of research in Tourette syndrome. Behav Neurol 2013;27(1):139–42.

International Review of Neurobiology 2013;112

Martino D, Cavanna AE. The metamorphoses of Gilles de la Tourette syndrome. Int Rev Neurobiol 2013;112:xv–xx.

Martino D, Madhusudan N, Zis P, Cavanna AE. An introduction to the clinical phenomenology of Tourette syndrome. Int Rev Neurobiol 2013;112:1–32.

Neuner I, Schneider F, Shah NJ. Functional neuroanatomy of tics. Int Rev Neurobiol 2013;112:35–71.

Segura B, Strafella AP. Functional imaging of dopaminergic neurotransmission in Tourette syndrome. Int Rev Neurobiol 2013;112:73–93.

Udvardi PT, Nespoli E, Rizzo F, Hengerer B, Ludolph AG. Nondopaminergic neurotransmission in the pathophysiology of Tourette syndrome. Int Rev Neurobiol 2013;112:95–130.

Palminteri S, Pessiglione M. Reinforcement learning and Tourette syndrome. Int Rev Neurobiol 2013;112:131–53.

Paschou P, Fernandez TV, Sharp F, Heiman GA, Hoekstra PJ. Genetic susceptibility and neurotransmitters in Tourette syndrome. Int Rev Neurobiol 2013;112:155–77.

McCairn KW, Isoda M. Pharmacological animal models of tic disorders. Int Rev Neurobiol 2013;112:179–209.

Macrì S, Onori MP, Roessner V, Laviola G. Animal models recapitulating the multifactorial origin of Tourette syndrome. Int Rev Neurobiol 2013;112:211–37.

Martino D, Macerollo A, Leckman JF. Neuroendocrine aspects of Tourette syndrome. Int Rev Neurobiol 2013;112:239–79.

Mogwitz S, Buse J, Ehrlich S, Roessner V. Clinical pharmacology of dopamine-modulating agents in Tourette's syndrome. Int Rev Neurobiol 2013;112:281–349.

Hartmann A. Clinical pharmacology of nondopaminergic drugs in Tourette syndrome. Int Rev Neurobiol 2013;112:351–72.

Cavanna AE, Nani A. Antiepileptic drugs and Tourette syndrome. Int Rev Neurobiol 2013;112:373–89.

Neri V, Cardona F. Clinical pharmacology of comorbid obsessive-compulsive disorder in Tourette syndrome. Int Rev Neurobiol 2013;112:391–414.

Rizzo R, Gulisano M. Clinical pharmacology of comorbid attention deficit hyperactivity disorder in Tourette syndrome. Int Rev Neurobiol 2013;112:415–44.

Termine C, Selvini C, Rossi G, Balottin U. Emerging treatment strategies in Tourette syndrome: What's in the pipeline? Int Rev Neurobiol 2013;112:445–80.

Madruga-Garrido M, Mir P. Tics and other stereotyped movements as side effects of pharmacological treatment. Int Rev Neurobiol 2013;112:481–94.

Neuroscience and Biobehavioral Reviews 2013;37(6)

Martino D, Laviola G. The multifaceted nature of Tourette syndrome: Pre-clinical, clinical and therapeutic issues. Neurosci Biobehav Rev 2013;37(6):993–6.

Cohen SC, Leckman JF, Bloch MH. Clinical assessment of Tourette syndrome and tic disorders. Neurosci Biobehav Rev 2013;37(6):997–1007.

Cavanna AE, Rickards HE. The psychopathological spectrum of Gilles de la Tourette syndrome. Neurosci Biobehav Rev 2013;37(6):1008–15.

Jung J, Jackson SR, Parkinson A, Jackson GM. Cognitive control over motor output in Tourette syndrome. Neurosci Biobehav Rev 2013;37(6):1016–25.

Paschou P. The genetic basis of Gilles de la Tourette syndrome. Neurosci Biobehav Rev 2013;37(6):1026–39.

Hoekstra PJ, Dietrich A, Edwards MJ, Elamin I, Martino D. Environmental factors in Tourette syndrome. Neurosci Biobehav Rev 2013;37(6):1040–9.

Ganos C, Roessner V, Münchau A. The functional anatomy of Gilles de la Tourette syndrome. Neurosci Biobehav Rev 2013;37(6):1050–62.

Priori A, Giannicola G, Rosa M, Marceglia S, Servello D, Sassi M, Porta M. Deep brain electrophysiological recordings provide clues to the pathophysiology of Tourette syndrome. Neurosci Biobehav Rev 2013;37(6):1063–8.

Buse J, Schoenefeld K, Münchau A, Roessner V. Neuromodulation in Tourette syndrome: Dopamine and beyond. Neurosci Biobehav Rev 2013;37(6):1069–84.

Macrì S, Proietti Onori M, Laviola G. Theoretical and practical considerations behind the use of laboratory animals for the study of Tourette syndrome. Neurosci Biobehav Rev 2013;37(6):1085–100.

Bronfeld M, Israelashvili M, Bar-Gad I. Pharmacological animal models of Tourette syndrome. Neurosci Biobehav Rev 2013;37(6):1101–19.

Hornig M, Lipkin WI. Immune-mediated animal models of Tourette syndrome. Neurosci Biobehav Rev 2013;37(6):1120–38.

Amitai N, Weber M, Swerdlow NR, Sharp RF, Breier MR, Halberstadt AL, Young JW. A novel visuospatial priming task for rats with relevance to Tourette syndrome and modulation of dopamine levels. Neurosci Biobehav Rev 2013;37(6):1139–49.

Hartmann A, Worbe Y. Pharmacological treatment of Gilles de la Tourette syndrome. Neurosci Biobehav Rev 2013;37(6):1157–61.

Weisman H, Qureshi IA, Leckman JF, Scahill L, Bloch MH. Systematic review: Pharmacological treatment of tic disorders – efficacy of antipsychotic and alpha-2 adrenergic agonist agents. Neurosci Biobehav Rev 2013;37(6):1162–71.

van de Griendt JM, Verdellen CW, van Dijk MK, Verbraak MJ. Behavioural treatment of tics: habit reversal and exposure with response prevention. Neurosci Biobehav Rev 2013;37(6):1172–7.

Müller-Vahl KR. Surgical treatment of Tourette syndrome. Neurosci Biobehav Rev 2013;37(6):1178–85.

Journal of Obsessive-Compulsive and Related Disorders 2014;3(4)

Black KJ, Jankovic J, Hershey T, McNaught KS, Mink JW, Walkup J. Progress in research on Tourette syndrome. J Obsessive-Compulsive Related Disord 2014;3(4):359–62.

Eddy CM, Cavanna AE. Tourette syndrome and obsessive compulsive disorder: Compulsivity along the continuum. J Obsessive-Compulsive Related Disord 2014;3(4):363–71.

Leckman JF, King RA, Bloch MH. Clinical features of Tourette syndrome and tic disorders. J Obsessive-Compulsive Related Disord 2014;3(4):372–9.

Pauls DL, Fernandez TV, Mathews CA, State MW, Scharf JM. The inheritance of Tourette disorder: A review. J Obsessive-Compulsive Related Disord 2014;3(4):380–5.

Church JA, Schlaggar BL. Pediatric Tourette syndrome: Insights from recent neuroimaging studies. J Obsessive-Compulsive Related Disord 2014;3(4):386–93.

Scahill L, Specht M, Page C. The prevalence of tic disorders and clinical characteristics in children. J Obsessive-Compulsive Related Disord 2014;3(4):394–400.

Visser-Vandewalle V, Huys D, Neuner I, Zrinzo L, Okun MS, Kuhn J. Deep brain stimulation for Tourette syndrome: The current state of the field. J Obsessive-Compulsive Related Disord 2014;3(4):401–6.

Gilbert DL, Jankovic J. Pharmacological treatment of Tourette syndrome. J Obsessive-Compulsive Related Disord 2014;3(4):407–14.

Capriotti MR, Himle MB, Woods DW. Behavioral treatments for Tourette syndrome. J Obsessive-Compulsive Related Disord 2014;3(4):415–20.

Children's Health Care 2015;44(3)

Rudy BM, Lewin AB, Storch EA. Introduction to the special issue: Considerations of the effects of extra-symptom variables among youth with chronic tic disorders and Tourette's syndrome. Children's Health Care 2015;44(3):199–204.

Capriotti MR, Piacentini JC, Himle MB, Ricketts EJ, Espil FM, Lee HJ, Turkel JE, Woods DW. Assessing environmental consequences of ticcing in youth with chronic tic disorders: The tic accommodation and reactions scale. Children's Health Care 2015;44(3):205–20.

Eaton CK, Gutierrez-Colina AM, Lee JL, Blount RL. Predictors of experiences and attitudes at a summer camp for children and adolescents with Tourette syndrome. Children's Health Care 2015;44(3):221–34.

Rozenman M, Johnson OE, Chang SW, Woods DW, Walkup JT, Wilhelm S, Peterson A, Scahill L, Piacentini J.

Relationships between premonitory urge and anxiety in youth with chronic tic disorders. Children's Health Care 2015;44(3):235–48.

Ramanujam K, Himle MB, Hayes LP, Woods DW, Scahill L, Sukhodolsky DG, Wilhelm S, Deckersbach T, Peterson AL, Specht M, Walkup JT, Chang SW, Piacentini J. Clinical correlates and predictors of caregiver strain in children with chronic tic disorders. Children's Health Care 2015;44(3):249–63.

Cavanna AE, Selvini C, Luoni C, Eddy CM, Ali F, Blangiardo R, Gagliardi E, Balottin U, Termine C. Measuring anger expression in young patients with Tourette syndrome. Children's Health Care 2015;44(3):264–76.

McGuire JF, Park JM, Wu MS, Lewin AB, Murphy TK, Storch EA. The impact of tic severity dimensions on impairment and quality of life among youth with chronic tic disorders. Children's Health Care 2015;44(3):277–92.

Nonaka M, Matsuda N, Kono T, Fujio M, Scahill L, Kano Y. Preliminary study of behavioral therapy for Tourette syndrome patients in Japan. Children's Health Care 2015;44(3):293–306.

Current Developmental Disorders Reports 2015;2(4)

Budman CL, Rosen M, Shad S. Fits, tantrums, and rages in TS and related disorders. Curr Develop Disord Rep 2015;2(4):273–84.

Hanks CE, Lewin AB, Mutch PJ, Storch EA, Murphy TK. Social deficits and autism spectrum disorders in Tourette's syndrome. Curr Develop Disord Rep 2015;2(4):285–92.

Coffey BJ. Complexities for assessment and treatment of co-occurring ADHD and tics. Curr Develop Disord Rep 2015;2(4):293–9.

Greene DJ, Schlaggar BL, Black KJ. Neuroimaging in Tourette syndrome: Research highlights from 2014–2015. Curr Develop Disord Rep 2015;2(4):300–8.

McGuire JF, Ricketts EJ, Piacentini J, Murphy TK, Storch EA, Lewin AB. Behavior therapy for tic disorders: An evidenced-based review and new directions for treatment research. Curr Develop Disord Rep 2015;2(4):309–17.

Movement Disorders 2015;30(9)

Tremblay L, Worbe Y, Thobois S, Sgambato-Faure V, Féger J. Selective dysfunction of basal ganglia subterritories: From movement to behavioral disorders. Mov Disord 2015;30 (9):1155–70.

Yael D, Vinner E, Bar-Gad I. Pathophysiology of tic disorders. Mov Disord 2015;30(9):1171–8.

Worbe Y, Lehericy S, Hartmann A. Neuroimaging of tic genesis: Present status and future perspectives. Mov Disord 2015;30 (9):1179–83.

Ganos C, Bongert J, Asmuss L, Martino D, Haggard P, Münchau A. The somatotopy of tic inhibition: Where and how much? Mov Disord 2015;30(9):1184–9.

Tinaz S, Malone P, Hallett M, Horovitz SG. Role of the right dorsal anterior insula in the urge to tic in Tourette syndrome. Mov Disord 2015;30(9):1190–7.

Ganos C, Garrido A, Navalpotro-Gómez I, Ricciardi L, Martino D, Edwards MJ, Tsakiris M, Haggard P, Bhatia KP. Premonitory urge to tic in Tourette's is associated with interoceptive awareness. Mov Disord 2015;30(9):1198–202.

Journal of Neuroscience Methods 2017;292

Bortolato M, Di Giovanni G. Editorial on special issue: Animal models of Tourette syndrome. J Neurosci Methods 2017;292:1.

Burton FH. Back to the future: Circuit-testing TS & OCD. J Neurosci Methods 2017;292:2–11.

Bortolato M, Pittenger C. Modeling tics in rodents: Conceptual challenges and paths forward. J Neurosci Methods 2017;292:12–19.

Vinner E, Israelashvili M, Bar-Gad I. Prolonged striatal disinhibition as a chronic animal model of tic disorders. J Neurosci Methods 2017;292:20–9.

Kreiss DS, De Deurwaerdère P. Purposeless oral activity induced by meta-chlorophenylpiperazine (m-CPP): Undefined tic-like behaviors? J Neurosci Methods 2017;292:30–6.

Fowler SC, Mosher LJ, Godar SC, Bortolato M. Assessment of gait and sensorimotor deficits in the D1CT-7 mouse model of Tourette syndrome. J Neurosci Methods 2017;292:37–44.

Roberts K, Hemmings AJ, McBride SD, Parker MO. Developing a 3-choice serial reaction time task for examining neural and cognitive function in an equine model. J Neurosci Methods 2017;292:45–52.

Bhakta SG, Young JW. The 5 choice continuous performance test (5 C-CPT): A novel tool to assess cognitive control across species. J Neurosci Methods 2017;292:53–60.

Current Developmental Disorders Reports 2018;5(2)

Grisolano LA. Tourette's from a neuropsychological perspective. Curr Develop Disord Rep 2018;5(2):89–94.

Kumar A, Duda L, Mainali G, Asghar S, Byler D. A comprehensive review of Tourette syndrome and complementary alternative medicine. Curr Develop Disord Rep 2018;5 (2):95–100.

Sharp AN, Singer HS. Standard, complementary, and future treatment options for tics. Curr Develop Disord Rep 2018;5(2):101–7.

Books

Meige H, Feindel E. Les tics et leur traitement. Paris: Masson 1902 (English version: Meige H, Feindel E. Tics and their treatment. Translated and edited with a critical appendix by Wilson SAK. London: Sidney Appleton 1907)

Meige H, Feindel E. The confessions of a victim to tic. In: Tics and their treatment. London: Sidney Appleton 1907; 1–24.

Meige H, Feindel E. Historical. In: Tics and their treatment. London: Sidney Appleton 1907; 25–35.

Meige H, Feindel E. The pathogeny of tic. In: Tics and their treatment. London: Sidney Appleton 1907; 36–73.

Meige H, Feindel E. The mental condition of tic subjects. In: Tics and their treatment. London: Sidney Appleton 1907; 74–95.

Meige H, Feindel E. The etiology of tics. In: Tics and their treatment. London: Sidney Appleton 1907; 96–107.

Meige H, Feindel E. Pathological anatomy. In: Tics and their treatment. London: Sidney Appleton 1907; 108–17.

Meige H, Feindel E. Study of the motor reaction. In: Tics and their treatment. London: Sidney Appleton 1907; 118–33.

Meige H, Feindel E. Accessory symptoms. In: Tics and their treatment. London: Sidney Appleton 1907; 134–41.

Meige H, Feindel E. The different tics. In: Tics and their treatment. London: Sidney Appleton 1907; 142–205.

Meige H, Feindel E. Tics of speech. In: Tics and their treatment. London: Sidney Appleton 1907; 206–20.

Meige H, Feindel E. The evolution of tics. In: Tics and their treatment. London: Sidney Appleton 1907; 221–35.

Meige H, Feindel E. Antagonistic gestures and stratagems. In: Tics and their treatment. London: Sidney Appleton 1907; 236–41.

Meige H, Feindel E. The complications of tics. In: Tics and their treatment. London: Sidney Appleton 1907; 242–4.

Meige H, Feindel E. The relation of tics to other pathological conditions. In: Tics and their treatment. London: Sidney Appleton 1907; 245–59.

Meige H, Feindel E. The distinctive features of tics. In: Tics and their treatment. London: Sidney Appleton 1907; 260–3.

Meige H, Feindel E. Diagnosis. In: Tics and their treatment. London: Sidney Appleton 1907; 264–92.

Meige H, Feindel E. Prognosis. In: Tics and their treatment. London: Sidney Appleton 1907; 293–7.

Meige H, Feindel E. The treatment of tics. In: Tics and their treatment. London: Sidney Appleton 1907; 298–314.

Meige H, Feindel E. Treatment by re-education. In: Tics and their treatment. London: Sidney Appleton 1907; 315–45.

Shapiro, A. K., Shapiro, E. S., Bruun, R. D., & Sweet, R. D. Gilles de la Tourette syndrome. New York: Raven Press 1978

Shapiro AK, Shapiro ES, Bruun RD, Sweet RD. Introduction. In: Gilles de la Tourette syndrome. New York: Raven Press 1978; 1–10.

Shapiro AK, Shapiro ES, Bruun RD, Sweet RD. History of tics and Tourette syndrome. In: Gilles de la Tourette syndrome. New York: Raven Press 1978; 11–82.

Shapiro AK, Shapiro ES, Bruun RD, Sweet RD. Samples, procedures, and hypotheses. In: Gilles de la Tourette syndrome. New York: Raven Press 1978; 83–90.

Shapiro AK, Shapiro ES, Bruun RD, Sweet RD. Demographic, family, birth, and developmental history. In: Gilles de la Tourette syndrome. New York: Raven Press 1978; 91–118.

Shapiro AK, Shapiro ES, Bruun RD, Sweet RD. Signs, symptoms, and clinical course. In: Gilles de la Tourette syndrome. New York: Raven Press 1978; 119–49.

Shapiro AK, Shapiro ES, Bruun RD, Sweet RD. Psychology. In: Gilles de la Tourette syndrome. New York: Raven Press 1978; 151–86.

Shapiro AK, Shapiro ES, Bruun RD, Sweet RD. Neurology. In: Gilles de la Tourette syndrome. New York: Raven Press 1978; 187–98.

Shapiro AK, Shapiro ES, Bruun RD, Sweet RD. Neural mechanisms in Tourette syndrome. In: Gilles de la Tourette syndrome. New York: Raven Press 1978; 199–221.

Shapiro AK, Shapiro ES, Bruun RD, Sweet RD. Electroencephalograms. In: Gilles de la Tourette syndrome. New York: Raven Press 1978; 223–38.

Shapiro AK, Shapiro ES, Bruun RD, Sweet RD. Differential diagnosis of tic syndromes and diagnostic nomenclature. In: Gilles de la Tourette syndrome. New York: Raven Press 1978; 239–57.

Shapiro AK, Shapiro ES, Bruun RD, Sweet RD. Genetics. In: Gilles de la Tourette syndrome. New York: Raven Press 1978; 259–69.

Shapiro AK, Shapiro ES, Bruun RD, Sweet RD. Studies of treatment. In: Gilles de la Tourette syndrome. New York: Raven Press 1978; 271–314.

Shapiro AK, Shapiro ES, Bruun RD, Sweet RD. Current treatment of Tourette syndrome. In: Gilles de la Tourette syndrome. New York: Raven Press 1978; 315–61.

Shapiro AK, Shapiro ES, Bruun RD, Sweet RD. Conclusions and research suggestions. In: Gilles de la Tourette syndrome. New York: Raven Press 1978; 363–75.

Kushner H. A cursing brain? The histories of Tourette syndrome. Cambridge, MA: Harvard University Press 1999

Kushner H. An elusive syndrome. In: A cursing brain? The histories of Tourette syndrome. Cambridge, MA: Harvard University Press 1999; 1–9.

Kushner H. The case of the cursing marquise. In: A cursing brain? The histories of Tourette syndrome. Cambridge, MA: Harvard University Press 1999; 10–25.

Kushner H. A disputed illness. In: A cursing brain? The histories of Tourette syndrome. Cambridge, MA: Harvard University Press 1999; 26–44.

Kushner H. The case of 'O.' and the emergence of psychoanalysis. In: A cursing brain? The histories of Tourette syndrome. Cambridge, MA: Harvard University Press 1999; 45–65.

Kushner H. Competing claims. In: A cursing brain? The histories of Tourette syndrome. Cambridge, MA: Harvard University Press 1999; 66–81.

Kushner H. The disappearance of tic illness. In: A cursing brain? The histories of Tourette syndrome. Cambridge, MA: Harvard University Press 1999; 82–98.

Kushner H. Margaret Mahler and the tic syndrome. In: A cursing brain? The histories of Tourette syndrome. Cambridge, MA: Harvard University Press 1999; 99–118.

Kushner H. Haloperidol and the persistence of the psychogenic frame. In: A cursing brain? The histories of Tourette syndrome. Cambridge, MA: Harvard University Press 1999; 119–43.

Kushner H. The French resistance. In: A cursing brain? The histories of Tourette syndrome. Cambridge, MA: Harvard University Press 1999; 144–64.

Kushner H. The triumph of the organic narrative. In: A cursing brain? The histories of Tourette syndrome. Cambridge, MA: Harvard University Press 1999; 165–93.

Kushner H. Clashing cultural conceptions. In: A cursing brain? The histories of Tourette syndrome. Cambridge, MA: Harvard University Press 1999; 194–212.

Kushner H. Clinical lessons. In: A cursing brain? The histories of Tourette syndrome. Cambridge, MA: Harvard University Press 1999; 213–22.

Kurlan R (Ed). Handbook of Tourette's syndrome and related tic and behavioral disorders. 2nd edn. New York: Marcel Dekker 2005

Fahn S. Motor and vocal tics. In: Kurlan R (Ed), Handbook of Tourette's syndrome and related tic and behavioral disorders. 2nd edn. New York: Marcel Dekker 2005; 1–14.

Pringsheim TM, Lang AE. Premonitory ("sensory") experiences. In: Kurlan R (Ed), Handbook of Tourette's syndrome and related tic and behavioral disorders. 2nd edn. New York: Marcel Dekker 2005; 15–22.

Bruun RD, Budman CL. The natural history of Gilles de la Tourette syndrome. In: Kurlan R (Ed), Handbook of Tourette's syndrome and related tic and behavioral disorders. 2nd edn. New York: Marcel Dekker 2005; 23–37.

Eapen V, Yakeley JW, Robertson MM. Obsessive-compulsive disorder and self-injurious behavior. In: Kurlan R (Ed), Handbook of Tourette's syndrome and related tic and behavioral disorders. 2nd edn. New York: Marcel Dekker 2005; 39–88.

Palumbo D. New directions in the treatment of comorbid attention deficit hyperactivity disorder and Tourette's syndrome. In: Kurlan R (Ed), Handbook of Tourette's syndrome and related tic and behavioral disorders. 2nd edn. New York: Marcel Dekker 2005; 89–108.

Coffey BJ, Frisone D, Gianini L. Anxiety and other comorbid emotional disorders. In: Kurlan R (Ed), Handbook of Tourette's syndrome and related tic and behavioral disorders. 2nd edn. New York: Marcel Dekker 2005; 109–26.

Budman CL, Rockmore L, Bruun RD. Aggressive symptoms and Tourette's syndrome. In: Kurlan R (Ed), Handbook of Tourette's syndrome and related tic and behavioral disorders. 2nd edn. New York: Marcel Dekker 2005; 127–54.

Erenberg G. Primary tic disorders. In: Kurlan R (Ed), Handbook of Tourette's syndrome and related tic and behavioral disorders. 2nd edn. New York: Marcel Dekker 2005; 155–72.

Jankovic J, Kwak C. Tics in other neurological disorders. In: Kurlan R (Ed), Handbook of Tourette's syndrome and related tic and behavioral disorders. 2nd edn. New York: Marcel Dekker 2005; 173–94.

Anderson KE, Weiner WJ. Drug-induced tics. In: Kurlan R (Ed), Handbook of Tourette's syndrome and related tic and behavioral disorders. 2nd edn. New York: Marcel Dekker 2005; 195–214.

Kurlan R, McDermott MP. Rating tic severity. In: Kurlan R (Ed), Handbook of Tourette's syndrome and related tic and behavioral disorders. 2nd edn. New York: Marcel Dekker 2005; 215–36.

Como PG. Neuropsychological function in Tourette's syndrome. In: Kurlan R (Ed), Handbook of Tourette's syndrome and related tic and behavioral disorders. 2nd edn. New York: Marcel Dekker 2005; 237–52.

Mink JW. Basal ganglia circuits and thalamocortical outputs. In: Kurlan R (Ed), Handbook of Tourette's syndrome and related tic and behavioral disorders. 2nd edn. New York: Marcel Dekker 2005; 253–72.

Singer HS, Minzer K. Neurobiological issues in Tourette's syndrome. In: Kurlan R (Ed), Handbook of Tourette's syndrome and related tic and behavioral disorders. 2nd edn. New York: Marcel Dekker 2005; 273–318.

McMahon WM, Johnson M. Infection and autoimmune factors in Tourette's and related disorders. In: Kurlan R (Ed), Handbook of Tourette's syndrome and related tic and behavioral disorders. 2nd edn. New York: Marcel Dekker 2005; 319–50.

Feigin A, Eidelberg D. Imaging in Tourette's syndrome. In: Kurlan R (Ed), Handbook of Tourette's syndrome and related tic and behavioral disorders. 2nd edn. New York: Marcel Dekker 2005; 351–63.

Rosario-Campos MC, Pauls DL. The inheritance pattern. In: Kurlan R (Ed), Handbook of Tourette's syndrome and related tic and behavioral disorders. 2nd edn. New York: Marcel Dekker 2005; 365–78.

Barr CL. Progress in gene localization. In: Kurlan R (Ed), Handbook of Tourette's syndrome and related tic and behavioral disorders. 2nd edn. New York: Marcel Dekker 2005; 379–98.

Tanner CM. Epidemiology of Tourette's syndrome. In: Kurlan R (Ed), Handbook of Tourette's syndrome and related tic and behavioral disorders. 2nd edn. New York: Marcel Dekker 2005; 399–410.

Goetz CG, Horn S. The treatment of tics. In: Kurlan R (Ed), Handbook of Tourette's syndrome and related tic and behavioral disorders. 2nd edn. New York: Marcel Dekker 2005; 411–26.

King RA, Findley D, Scahill L, Vitulano LA, Leckman JF. Obsessive-compulsive disorder in Tourette's syndrome: Treatment and other considerations. In: Kurlan R (Ed), Handbook of Tourette's syndrome and related tic and behavioral disorders. 2nd edn. New York: Marcel Dekker 2005; 427–54.

Brown L, Dure LS. The treatment of comorbid attention-deficit disorder and Tourette's syndrome. In: Kurlan R (Ed), Handbook of Tourette's syndrome and related tic and behavioral disorders. 2nd edn. New York: Marcel Dekker 2005; 455–66.

van der Linden C, Colle H, Foncke EMJ, Bruggeman R. The neurosurgical treatment of Tourette's syndrome. In: Kurlan R (Ed), Handbook of Tourette's syndrome and related tic and behavioral disorders. 2nd edn. New York: Marcel Dekker 2005; 467–74.

Conneally PM. Genetic counseling. In: Kurlan R (Ed), Handbook of Tourette's syndrome and related tic and behavioral disorders. 2nd edn. New York: Marcel Dekker 2005; 475–80.

Leckman JF, Cohen DJ. The child and adolescent with Tourette's syndrome: Clinical perspectives on phenomenology. In: Kurlan R (Ed), Handbook of Tourette's syndrome and related tic and behavioral disorders. 2nd edn. New York: Marcel Dekker 2005; 481–504.

Sacks O. Tourette's syndrome: A human condition. In: Kurlan R (Ed), Handbook of Tourette's syndrome and related tic and behavioral disorders. 2nd edn. New York: Marcel Dekker 2005; 505–10.

Levi-Pearl S. The Tourette Syndrome Association, Inc. In: Kurlan R (Ed), Handbook of Tourette's syndrome and related tic and behavioral disorders. 2nd edn. New York: Marcel Dekker 2005; 511–17.

Woods DW, Piacentini J, Walkup JT (Eds). Treating Tourette syndrome and tic disorders: A guide for practitioners. New York: Guilford Press 2007

Woods DW, Piacentini JC, Walkup JT. Introduction to clinical management of

Tourette syndrome. In: Woods DW, Piacentini J, Walkup JT (Eds). Treating Tourette syndrome and tic disorders: A guide for practitioners. New York: Guilford Press 2007; 1–5.

Piacentini JC, Pearlman AJ, Peris TS. Characteristics of Tourette syndrome. In: Woods DW, Piacentini J, Walkup JT (Eds). Treating Tourette syndrome and tic disorders: A guide for practitioners. New York: Guilford Press 2007; 9–21.

Woods DW, Piacentini JC, Himle MB. Assessment of tic disorders. In: Woods DW, Piacentini J, Walkup JT (Eds). Treating Tourette syndrome and tic disorders: A guide for practitioners. New York: Guilford Press 2007; 22–38.

Scahill L, Sukhodolsky DG, King RA. Assessment of co-occurring psychiatric conditions in tic disorders. In: Woods DW, Piacentini J, Walkup JT (Eds). Treating Tourette syndrome and tic disorders: A guide for practitioners. New York: Guilford Press 2007; 38–57.

Leary J, Reimschisel T, Singer HS. Genetic and neurobiological bases for Tourette syndrome. In: Woods DW, Piacentini J, Walkup JT (Eds). Treating Tourette syndrome and tic disorders: A guide for practitioners. New York: Guilford Press 2007; 58–84.

Chang S. Neurocognitive factors in Tourette syndrome. In: Woods DW, Piacentini J, Walkup JT (Eds). Treating Tourette syndrome and tic disorders: A guide for practitioners. New York: Guilford Press 2007; 85–109.

Harrison JN, Schneider B, Walkup JT. Medical management of Tourette syndrome and co-occurring conditions. In: Woods DW, Piacentini J, Walkup JT (Eds). Treating Tourette syndrome and tic disorders: A guide for practitioners. New York: Guilford Press 2007; 113–53.

Peterson AL. Psychosocial management of tics and intentional repetitive behaviors associated with Tourette syndrome. In: Woods DW, Piacentini J, Walkup JT (Eds). Treating Tourette syndrome and tic disorders: A guide for practitioners. New York: Guilford Press 2007; 154–84.

Buhlmann U, Deckersbach T, Cook L, Wilhelm S. Psychosocial management of comorbid internalizing disorders in persons with Tourette syndrome. In: Woods DW, Piacentini J, Walkup JT (Eds). Treating

Tourette syndrome and tic disorders: A guide for practitioners. New York: Guilford Press 2007; 185–98.

Sukhodolsky DG, Scahill L. Disruptive behavior in persons with Tourette syndrome: Phenomenology, assessment, and treatment. In: Woods DW, Piacentini J, Walkup JT (Eds). Treating Tourette syndrome and tic disorders: A guide for practitioners. New York: Guilford Press 2007; 199–221.

Ginsburg GS, Newman Kingery J. Management of familial issues in persons with Tourette syndrome. In: Woods DW, Piacentini J, Walkup JT (Eds). Treating Tourette syndrome and tic disorders: A guide for practitioners. New York: Guilford Press 2007; 225–41.

Kepley HO, Conners S. Management of learning and school difficulties in children with Tourette syndrome. In: Woods DW, Piacentini J, Walkup JT (Eds). Treating Tourette syndrome and tic disorders: A guide for practitioners. New York: Guilford Press 2007; 242–64.

Woods DW, Marcks BA, Flessner CA. Management of social and occupational difficulties in persons with Tourette syndrome. In: Woods DW, Piacentini J, Walkup JT (Eds). Treating Tourette syndrome and tic disorders: A guide for practitioners. New York: Guilford Press 2007; 265–77.

Robertson MM, Cavanna AE. Tourette syndrome: The facts. 2nd edn. Oxford: Oxford University Press 2008

Robertson MM, Cavanna AE. Introducing three cases. In: Tourette syndrome: The facts. 2nd edn. Oxford: Oxford University Press 2008; 1–12.

Robertson MM, Cavanna AE. What is Tourette syndrome? In: Tourette syndrome: The facts. 2nd edn. Oxford: Oxford University Press 2008; 13–16.

Robertson MM, Cavanna AE. How common is Tourette syndrome? In: Tourette syndrome: The facts. 2nd edn. Oxford: Oxford University Press 2008; 17–20.

Robertson MM, Cavanna AE. How is the diagnosis made? In: Tourette syndrome: The facts. 2nd edn. Oxford: Oxford University Press 2008; 21–9.

Robertson MM, Cavanna AE. What other disorders can be mistaken for Tourette syndrome? In: Tourette syndrome: The facts. 2nd edn. Oxford: Oxford University Press 2008; 31–4.

Robertson MM, Cavanna AE. Can people with Tourette syndrome also develop other conditions? In: Tourette syndrome: The facts. 2nd edn. Oxford: Oxford University Press 2008; 35–41.

Robertson MM, Cavanna AE. Will I have Tourette syndrome forever? In: Tourette syndrome: The facts. 2nd edn. Oxford: Oxford University Press 2008; 43–7.

Robertson MM, Cavanna AE. Coping with the news of the diagnosis of Tourette syndrome. In: Tourette syndrome: The facts. 2nd edn. Oxford: Oxford University Press 2008; 49–59.

Robertson MM, Cavanna AE. Is there more than one type of Tourette syndrome? In: Tourette syndrome: The facts. 2nd edn. Oxford: Oxford University Press 2008; 61–5.

Robertson MM, Cavanna AE. What causes Tourette syndrome? In: Tourette syndrome: The facts. 2nd edn. Oxford: Oxford University Press 2008; 67–73.

Robertson MM, Cavanna AE. Which therapies are most useful for Tourette syndrome? In: Tourette syndrome: The facts. 2nd edn. Oxford: Oxford University Press 2008; 75–81.

Robertson MM, Cavanna AE. Education, employment, and empowerment. In: Tourette syndrome: The facts. 2nd edn. Oxford: Oxford University Press 2008; 83–106.

Robertson MM, Cavanna AE. Famous or successful people who have had Tourette syndrome. In: Tourette syndrome: The facts. 2nd edn. Oxford: Oxford University Press 2008; 107–26.

Walkup JT, Mink JW, McNaught K (Eds). A family's guide to Tourette syndrome. Bloomington, IN: iUniverse 2012

Jankovic J. Introduction. In: Walkup JT, Mink JW, McNaught K (Eds). A family's guide to Tourette syndrome. Bloomington, IN: iUniverse 2012; 1–7.

Leckman JF, Bloch MH, King RA. The diagnosis of Tourette syndrome. In: Walkup JT, Mink JW, McNaught K (Eds). A family's guide to Tourette syndrome. Bloomington, IN: iUniverse 2012; 8–23.

Coffey BJ, Zwilling A. Psychiatric conditions associated with Tourette syndrome. In: Walkup JT, Mink JW, McNaught K (Eds). A family's guide to Tourette syndrome. Bloomington, IN: iUniverse 2012; 24–47.

Budman CL, Witkin J. Problems with anger, aggression, and impulse control in Tourette syndrome. In: Walkup JT, Mink JW, McNaught K (Eds). A family's guide to Tourette syndrome. Bloomington, IN: iUniverse 2012; 48–66.

Scahill L. How common is Tourette syndrome in children? In: Walkup JT, Mink JW, McNaught K (Eds). A family's guide to Tourette syndrome. Bloomington, IN: iUniverse 2012; 67–72.

Mink JW. The causes of TS and changes that occur in the brain. In: Walkup JT, Mink JW, McNaught K (Eds). A family's guide to Tourette syndrome. Bloomington, IN: iUniverse 2012; 73–81.

Scharf JM, Mathews CA. Inheritance, genes, and TS. In: Walkup JT, Mink JW, McNaught K (Eds). A family's guide to Tourette syndrome. Bloomington, IN: iUniverse 2012; 82–96.

Murphy T. Pediatric autoimmune neuropsychiatric disorders associated with streptococcal infection (PANDAS) and Tourette syndrome. In: Walkup JT, Mink JW, McNaught K (Eds). A family's guide to Tourette syndrome. Bloomington, IN: iUniverse 2012; 97–109.

Gilbert DL. Drug treatments for Tourette syndrome and co-morbid disorders. In: Walkup JT, Mink JW, McNaught K (Eds). A family's guide to Tourette syndrome. Bloomington, IN: iUniverse 2012; 110–24.

Muelly ER, Berlin CM Jr. Tourette syndrome, pregnancy and breastfeeding. In: Walkup JT, Mink JW, McNaught K (Eds). A family's guide to Tourette syndrome. Bloomington, IN: iUniverse 2012; 125–34.

Capriotti MR, Espil FM, Woods DW. Behavior therapy. In: Walkup JT, Mink JW, McNaught K (Eds). A family's guide to Tourette syndrome. Bloomington, IN: iUniverse 2012; 135–44.

Okun MS, Ward H, Malaty I, Ricciuti N, Hill C, Foote KD. Deep brain stimulation for

Tourette syndrome. In: Walkup JT, Mink JW, McNaught K (Eds). A family's guide to Tourette syndrome. Bloomington, IN: iUniverse 2012; 145–54.

Kompoliti K. Complementary and alternative therapies. In: Walkup JT, Mink JW, McNaught K (Eds). A family's guide to Tourette syndrome. Bloomington, IN: iUniverse 2012; 155–70.

Robertson MM. The psychological aspects of Tourette syndrome: A family guide and perspective. In: Walkup JT, Mink JW, McNaught K (Eds). A family's guide to Tourette syndrome. Bloomington, IN: iUniverse 2012; 171–92.

Zinner SH, Erdie-Lalena C. Living with Tourette syndrome. In: Walkup JT, Mink JW, McNaught K (Eds). A family's guide to Tourette syndrome. Bloomington, IN: iUniverse 2012; 193–208.

Fantle Shimberg E. Parenting a child with Tourette syndrome. In: Walkup JT, Mink JW, McNaught K (Eds). A family's guide to Tourette syndrome. Bloomington, IN: iUniverse 2012; 209–21.

McNaught K. History and research into Tourette syndrome. In: Walkup JT, Mink JW, McNaught K (Eds). A family's guide to Tourette syndrome. Bloomington, IN: iUniverse 2012; 222–8.

McNaught K. Frequently asked questions and answers about Tourette syndrome. In: Walkup JT, Mink JW, McNaught K (Eds). A family's guide to Tourette syndrome. Bloomington, IN: iUniverse 2012; 229–72.

Martino D, Leckman JF (Eds). Tourette syndrome. Oxford: Oxford University Press 2013

Leckman JF, Bloch MH, Sukhodolsky DG, Scahill L, King RA. Phenomenology of tics and sensory urges: The self under siege. In: Martino D, Leckman JF (Eds). Tourette syndrome. Oxford: Oxford University Press 2013; 3–25.

Rothenberger A, Roessner V. The phenomenology of attention-deficit/hyperactivity disorder in Tourette syndrome. In: Martino D, Leckman JF (Eds). Tourette syndrome. Oxford: Oxford University Press 2013; 26–49.

Ferrao YA, Gomes de Alvarenga P, Hounie AG, de Mathis MA, Conceição de Rosario M, Miguel EC. The phenomenology of obsessive-compulsive symptoms in Tourette syndrome. In: Martino D, Leckman JF (Eds). Tourette syndrome. Oxford: Oxford University Press 2013; 50–73.

Cath D, Ludolph A. Other psychiatric comorbidities in Tourette syndrome. In: Martino D, Leckman JF (Eds). Tourette syndrome. Oxford: Oxford University Press 2013; 74–106.

Bloch MH. Clinical course and adult outcome in Tourette syndrome. In: Martino D, Leckman JF (Eds). Tourette syndrome. Oxford: Oxford University Press 2013; 107–20.

Scahill L, Dalsgaard S. The prevalence of Tourette syndrome and its relationship to clinical features. In: Martino D, Leckman JF (Eds). Tourette syndrome. Oxford: Oxford University Press 2013; 121–33.

Fernandez TV, State MW. Genetic susceptibility in Tourette syndrome. In: Martino D, Leckman JF (Eds). Tourette syndrome. Oxford: Oxford University Press 2013; 137–55.

Hoekstra PJ. Perinatal adversities and Tourette syndrome. In: Martino D, Leckman JF (Eds). Tourette syndrome. Oxford: Oxford University Press 2013; 156–67.

Murphy TK. Infections and tic disorders. In: Martino D, Leckman JF (Eds). Tourette syndrome. Oxford: Oxford University Press 2013; 168–201.

Vaccarino FM, Kataoka Y, Lennington J. Cellular and molecular pathology in Tourette syndrome. In: Martino D, Leckman JF (Eds). Tourette syndrome. Oxford: Oxford University Press 2013; 205–20.

Orth M. Electrophysiology in Tourette syndrome. In: Martino D, Leckman JF (Eds). Tourette syndrome. Oxford: Oxford University Press 2013; 221–37.

Greene DJ, Black KJ, Schlaggar BL. Neurobiology and functional anatomy of tic disorders. In: Martino D, Leckman JF (Eds). Tourette syndrome. Oxford: Oxford University Press 2013; 238–75.

Singer HS. The neurochemistry of Tourette syndrome. In: Martino D, Leckman JF (Eds). Tourette syndrome. Oxford: Oxford University Press 2013; 276–300.

Martino D. Immunity and stress response in Tourette syndrome. In: Martino D, Leckman JF (Eds). Tourette syndrome. Oxford: Oxford University Press 2013; 301–28.

McCairn KW, Imamura Y, Isoda M. Animal models of tics. In: Martino D, Leckman JF (Eds). Tourette syndrome. Oxford: Oxford University Press 2013; 329–58.

Robertson MM, Eapen V. Whither the relationship between etiology and phenotype in Tourette syndrome? In: Martino D, Leckman JF (Eds). Tourette syndrome. Oxford: Oxford University Press 2013; 361–94.

Kurlan R. The differential diagnosis of tic disorders. In: Martino D, Leckman JF (Eds). Tourette syndrome. Oxford: Oxford University Press 2013; 395–401.

King RA, Landeros-Weisenberger A. Comprehensive assessment strategies. In: Martino D, Leckman JF (Eds). Tourette syndrome. Oxford: Oxford University Press 2013; 402–10.

Cavanna AE, Piedad JCP. Clinical rating instruments in Tourette syndrome. In: Martino D, Leckman JF (Eds). Tourette syndrome. Oxford: Oxford University Press 2013; 411–38.

Murphy T, Eddy C. Neuropsychological Assessment in Tourette Syndrome. In: Martino D, Leckman JF (Eds). Tourette syndrome. Oxford: Oxford University Press 2013; 439–67.

Sukhodolsky DG, Eicher VW, Leckman JF. Social and adaptive functioning in Tourette syndrome. In: Martino D, Leckman JF (Eds). Tourette syndrome. Oxford: Oxford University Press 2013; 468–84.

Lebowitz ER, Scahill L. Psychoeducational interventions: What every parent and family member needs to know. In: Martino D, Leckman JF (Eds). Tourette syndrome. Oxford: Oxford University Press 2013; 487–502.

Capriotti MR, Woods DW. Cognitive-behavioral treatment for tics. In: Martino D, Leckman JF (Eds). Tourette syndrome. Oxford: Oxford University Press 2013; 503–23.

Roessner V, Rothenberger A. Pharmacological treatment of tics. In: Martino D, Leckman JF (Eds). Tourette syndrome. Oxford: Oxford University Press 2013; 524–52.

Cardona F, Rizzo R. Treatment of psychiatric comorbidities in Tourette syndromes. In: Martino D, Leckman JF (Eds). Tourette syndrome. Oxford: Oxford University Press 2013; 553–82.

Porta M, Sassi M, Servello D. Surgical treatment of Tourette syndrome. In: Martino D, Leckman JF (Eds). Tourette syndrome. Oxford: Oxford University Press 2013; 583–604.

Zolovska B, Coffey B. Alternative treatments in Tourette syndrome. In: Martino D, Leckman JF (Eds). Tourette syndrome. Oxford: Oxford University Press 2013; 605–19.

Müller-Vahl K. Information and social support for patients and families. In: Martino D, Leckman JF (Eds). Tourette syndrome. Oxford: Oxford University Press 2013; 623–35.

Pruitt SK, Packer LE. Information and support for educators. In: Martino D, Leckman JF (Eds). Tourette syndrome. Oxford: Oxford University Press 2013; 636–55.

Roper L, Hollenbeck P, Rickards H. Tourette syndrome support organizations around the world. In: Martino D, Leckman JF (Eds). Tourette syndrome. Oxford: Oxford University Press 2013; 656–66.

Freeman R. Tics and Tourette syndrome: Key clinical perspectives. London: Mac Keith Press 2015

Freeman R. Introduction. In: Tics and Tourette syndrome: Key clinical perspectives. London: Mac Keith Press 2015; 1–7.

Freeman R. Diagnosis and definitions. In: Tics and Tourette syndrome: Key clinical perspectives. London: Mac Keith Press 2015; 8–24.

Freeman R. Presentation to clinicians. In: Tics and Tourette syndrome: Key clinical perspectives. London: Mac Keith Press 2015; 25–33.

Freeman R. Prevalence and epidemiology. In: Tics and Tourette syndrome: Key clinical perspectives. London: Mac Keith Press 2015; 34–6.

Freeman R. Etiology. In: Tics and Tourette syndrome: Key clinical perspectives. London: Mac Keith Press 2015; 37–42.

Freeman R. Clinical course and prognosis. In: Tics and Tourette syndrome: Key clinical perspectives. London: Mac Keith Press 2015; 43–7.

Freeman R. Phenomenology and social consequences. In: Tics and Tourette syndrome: Key clinical perspectives. London: Mac Keith Press 2015; 48–58.

Freeman R. The lived experience. In: Tics and Tourette syndrome: Key clinical perspectives. London: Mac Keith Press 2015; 59–61.

Freeman R. Functional ('conversion disorder' or 'psychogenic') tics. In: Tics and Tourette syndrome: Key clinical perspectives. London: Mac Keith Press 2015; 62–4.

Freeman R. Comorbid disorders and symptomatology. In: Tics and Tourette syndrome: Key clinical perspectives. London: Mac Keith Press 2015; 65–123.

Freeman R. Stereotypic movement disorder. In: Tics and Tourette syndrome: Key clinical perspectives. London: Mac Keith Press 2015; 124–44.

Freeman R. Symptoms and patterns. In: Tics and Tourette syndrome: Key clinical perspectives. London: Mac Keith Press 2015; 145–90.

Freeman R. Tics in other medical conditions. In: Tics and Tourette syndrome: Key clinical perspectives. London: Mac Keith Press 2015; 191–213.

Freeman R. Neuropsychology. In: Tics and Tourette syndrome: Key clinical perspectives. London: Mac Keith Press 2015; 214–15.

Freeman R. Interventions and treatment. In: Tics and Tourette syndrome: Key clinical perspectives. London: Mac Keith Press 2015; 216–39.

Freeman R. Working with schools. In: Tics and Tourette syndrome: Key clinical perspectives. London: Mac Keith Press 2015; 240–5.

Freeman R. Working with families. In: Tics and Tourette syndrome: Key clinical perspectives. London: Mac Keith Press 2015; 246–55.

Freeman R. Peer relationships and teasing/bullying. In: Tics and Tourette syndrome: Key clinical perspectives. London: Mac Keith Press 2015; 256–9.

Freeman R. Controversies. In: Tics and Tourette syndrome: Key clinical perspectives. London: Mac Keith Press 2015; 260–3.

Freeman R. Refractory cases. In: Tics and Tourette syndrome: Key clinical perspectives. London: Mac Keith Press 2015; 264–5.

Freeman R. Service provision: A few considerations. In: Tics and Tourette syndrome: Key clinical perspectives. London: Mac Keith Press 2015; 266.

Freeman R. Support groups. In: Tics and Tourette syndrome: Key clinical perspectives. London: Mac Keith Press 2015; 267.

Freeman R. Tic disorders and the law. In: Tics and Tourette syndrome: Key clinical perspectives. London: Mac Keith Press 2015; 268–9.

Freeman R. Tourette syndrome, employment and insurance. In: Tics and Tourette syndrome: Key clinical perspectives. London: Mac Keith Press 2015; 270–1.

Freeman R. And now for something completely different. In: Tics and Tourette syndrome: Key clinical perspectives. London: Mac Keith Press 2015; 272–3.

Freeman R. Some problems tics can cause for others. In: Tics and Tourette syndrome: Key clinical perspectives. London: Mac Keith Press 2015; 274–9.

Freeman R. Coda. In: Tics and Tourette syndrome: Key clinical perspectives. London: Mac Keith Press 2015; 280–1.

Chowdhury U, Murphy T. Tic disorders: A guide for parents and professionals. London: Jessica Kingsley 2016

Chowdhury U, Murphy T. What are tic disorders? In: Tic disorders: A guide for parents and professionals. London: Jessica Kingsley 2016; 15–18.

Chowdhury U, Murphy T. Signs and symptoms. In: Tic disorders: A guide for parents and professionals. London: Jessica Kingsley 2016; 19–28.

Chowdhury U, Murphy T. Causes of tic disorders. In: Tic disorders: A guide for parents and professionals. London: Jessica Kingsley 2016; 29–39.

Chowdhury U, Murphy T. Working with schools. In: Tic disorders: A guide for parents and professionals. London: Jessica Kingsley 2016; 43–50.

Chowdhury U, Murphy T. Psychological management. In: Tic disorders: A guide for parents and professionals. London: Jessica Kingsley 2016; 51–61.

Chowdhury U, Murphy T. Medication. In: Tic disorders: A guide for parents and professionals. London: Jessica Kingsley 2016; 63–70.

Chowdhury U, Murphy T. Neurosurgery. In: Tic disorders: A guide for parents and professionals. London: Jessica Kingsley 2016; 71–5.

Chowdhury U, Murphy T. Not yet validated treatments. In: Tic disorders: A guide for parents and professionals. London: Jessica Kingsley 2016; 77–80.

Chowdhury U, Murphy T. Attention deficit hyperactivity disorder. In: Tic disorders: A guide for parents and professionals. London: Jessica Kingsley 2016; 83–90.

Chowdhury U, Murphy T. Obsessive compulsive disorder. In: Tic disorders: A guide for parents and professionals. London: Jessica Kingsley 2016; 91–7.

Chowdhury U, Murphy T. Depression. In: Tic disorders: A guide for parents and professionals. London: Jessica Kingsley 2016; 99–103.

Chowdhury U, Murphy T. Anxiety. In: Tic disorders: A guide for parents and professionals. London: Jessica Kingsley 2016; 105–10.

Chowdhury U, Murphy T. Autism spectrum disorder. In: Tic disorders: A guide for parents and professionals. London: Jessica Kingsley 2016; 111–14.

Chowdhury U, Murphy T. Specific learning difficulties. London: Jessica Kingsley 2016; 115–24.

Chowdhury U, Murphy T. Sleep. In: Tic disorders: A guide for parents and professionals. London: Jessica Kingsley 2016; 125–30.

Chowdhury U, Murphy T. Anger. In: Tic disorders: A guide for parents and professionals. London: Jessica Kingsley 2016; 131–9.

Chowdhury U, Murphy T. Adjusting to the diagnosis. In: Tic disorders: A guide for parents and professionals. London: Jessica Kingsley 2016; 143–51.

Chowdhury U, Murphy T. Dealing with behavioural problems. In: Tic disorders: A guide for parents and professionals. London: Jessica Kingsley 2016; 153–9.

Chowdhury U, Murphy T. Improving your child's self-esteem. In: Tic disorders: A guide for parents and professionals. London: Jessica Kingsley 2016; 161–6.

McGuire JF, Murphy TK, Piacentini J, Storch EA (Eds). The clinician's guide to treatment and management of youth with Tourette syndrome and tic disorders. San Diego, CA: Academic Press 2018

McGuire JF, Murphy TK, Piacentini J, Storch EA. Introduction to treatment and management of youth with Tourette disorders and tic disorders. In: McGuire JF, Murphy TK, Piacentini J, Storch EA (Eds). The clinician's guide to treatment and management of youth with Tourette syndrome and tic disorders. San Diego, CA: Academic Press 2018; 1–20.

Wu MS, McGuire JF. Psychoeducation about tic disorders and treatment. In: McGuire JF, Murphy TK, Piacentini J, Storch EA (Eds). The clinician's guide to treatment and management of youth with Tourette syndrome and tic disorders. San Diego, CA: Academic Press 2018; 21–42.

Ricketts EJ, Bauer CC. Habit reversal training for tics. In: McGuire JF, Murphy TK, Piacentini J, Storch EA (Eds). The clinician's guide to treatment and management of youth with Tourette syndrome and tic disorders. San Diego, CA: Academic Press 2018; 43–70.

Saggu BM, Shad S, Barnes AA, Budman CL. Pharmacological management of tic disorders in youth. In: McGuire JF, Murphy TK, Piacentini J, Storch EA (Eds). The clinician's guide to treatment and management of youth with Tourette syndrome and tic disorders. San Diego, CA: Academic Press 2018; 71–100.

Espil FM, Houghton DC. Cognitive restructuring about tics. In: McGuire JF, Murphy TK, Piacentini J, Storch EA (Eds). The clinician's guide to treatment and management of youth with Tourette syndrome and tic disorders. San Diego, CA: Academic Press 2018; 101–20.

Schreck MC, Conelea CA. Improving self-esteem for youth with Tourette syndrome and tic disorders. In: McGuire JF, Murphy TK, Piacentini J, Storch EA (Eds). The clinician's guide to treatment and management of youth with Tourette syndrome and tic disorders. San Diego, CA: Academic Press 2018; 121–38.

Dempsey J, Llorens AV, Fein R, Dempsey AG. Talking about tics with peers and coping in social interactions. In: McGuire JF, Murphy TK, Piacentini J, Storch EA (Eds). The clinician's guide to treatment and management of youth with Tourette syndrome and tic disorders. San Diego, CA: Academic Press 2018; 139–54.

Giordano K. Tourette's in the classroom: Support and guidance on education issues for clinicians. In: McGuire JF, Murphy TK, Piacentini J, Storch EA (Eds). The clinician's guide to treatment and management of youth with Tourette syndrome and tic disorders. San Diego, CA: Academic Press 2018; 155–76.

Nadeau JM, Hieneman M. Managing avoidance and accommodation of tics and related behaviors. In: McGuire JF, Murphy TK, Piacentini J, Storch EA (Eds). The clinician's guide to treatment and management of youth with Tourette syndrome and tic disorders. San Diego, CA: Academic Press 2018; 177–200.

Bennett SM, Beaumont R, Catarozoli C, Kushman AM. Problem-solving strategies to overcome common challenges associated with Tourette syndrome. In: McGuire JF, Murphy TK, Piacentini J, Storch EA (Eds). The clinician's guide to treatment and management of youth with Tourette syndrome and tic disorders. San Diego, CA: Academic Press 2018; 201–24.

Specht MW, Edwards KR, Perry-Parrish C, Amatya K. Brief trans-diagnostic parent training: A strengths-based, parent-centered treatment for youth with Tourette syndrome. In: McGuire JF, Murphy TK, Piacentini J, Storch EA (Eds). The clinician's guide to treatment and management of youth with Tourette syndrome and tic disorders. San Diego, CA: Academic Press 2018; 225–54.

Piasecka J, Bertschinger EJ, Tudor ME, Sukhodolsky DG. Assessing and treating emotion dysregulation and anger management. In: McGuire JF, Murphy TK, Piacentini J, Storch EA (Eds). The clinician's guide to treatment and management of youth with Tourette syndrome and tic disorders. San Diego, CA: Academic Press 2018; 255–78.

Reese HE. Mindfulness for tics. In: McGuire JF, Murphy TK, Piacentini J, Storch EA (Eds). The clinician's guide to treatment and management of youth with Tourette syndrome and tic disorders. San Diego, CA: Academic Press 2018; 279–300.

Himle MB, Wellen BCM, Hayes LP. Family issues associated with tics. In: McGuire JF, Murphy TK, Piacentini J, Storch EA (Eds). The clinician's guide to treatment and management of youth with Tourette syndrome and tic disorders. San Diego, CA: Academic Press 2018; 301–26.

Gera A, Kompoliti K. Promoting healthy behaviors. In: McGuire JF, Murphy TK, Piacentini J, Storch EA (Eds). The clinician's guide to treatment and management of youth with Tourette syndrome and tic disorders. San Diego, CA: Academic Press 2018; 327–46.

Selles RR, Jukes T, McConnell M, Stewart SE. Relapse prevention strategies and guidance on refractory cases. In: McGuire JF, Murphy TK, Piacentini J, Storch EA (Eds). The clinician's guide to treatment and management of youth with Tourette syndrome and tic disorders. San Diego, CA: Academic Press 2018; 347–74.

Walusinski O. Georges Gilles de la Tourette: Beyond the eponym. Oxford: Oxford University Press. 2018

Walusinski O. Georges Gilles de la Tourette (1857–1904): Origins and family life. In: Georges Gilles de la Tourette: Beyond the eponym. Oxford: Oxford University Press 2018; 3–18.

Walusinski O. Education, medical studies, medical practice. In: Georges Gilles de la Tourette: Beyond the eponym. Oxford: Oxford University Press 2018; 19–42.

Walusinski O. Secretary, colleague, and friend of Jean-Martin Charcot. In: Georges Gilles de la Tourette: Beyond the eponym. Oxford: Oxford University Press 2018; 43–69.

Walusinski O. The assassination attempt. Oxford: Oxford University Press 2018; 71–80.

Walusinski O. Glimpses of Gilles de la Tourette's personality: Hospital life and the Driout scandal. In: Georges Gilles de la Tourette: Beyond the eponym. Oxford: Oxford University Press 2018; 81–8.

Walusinski O. Chief physician for the 1900 World's Fair in Paris. In: Georges Gilles de la Tourette: Beyond the eponym. Oxford: Oxford University Press 2018; 89–99.

Walusinski O. EA sad end: Eclipse, twilight, and death. In: Georges Gilles de la Tourette: Beyond the eponym. Oxford: Oxford University Press 2018; 101–25.

Walusinski O. Doctoral thesis. In: Georges Gilles de la Tourette: Beyond the eponym. Oxford: Oxford University Press 2018; 129–43.

Walusinski O. Gilles de la Tourette syndrome. In: Georges Gilles de la Tourette: Beyond the eponym. Oxford: Oxford University Press 2018; 145–212.

Walusinski O. Vibratory medicine and therapeutic suspension techniques. In: Georges Gilles de la Tourette: Beyond the eponym. Oxford: Oxford University Press 2018; 213–46.

Walusinski O. Hypnotism and analogous states. In: Georges Gilles de la Tourette: Beyond the eponym. Oxford: Oxford University Press 2018; 247–75.

Walusinski O. Clinical and therapeutic treatise on hysteria: Hystérie normale. In: Georges Gilles de la Tourette: Beyond the eponym. Oxford: Oxford University Press 2018; 277–300.

Walusinski O. Clinical and therapeutic treatise on hysteria: Paroxysmic hysteria. In: Georges Gilles de la Tourette: Beyond the eponym. Oxford: Oxford University Press 2018; 301–33.

Walusinski O. Sœur Jeanne des Anges, supérieure des Ursulines de Loudun: A book by Gabriel Legué and Georges Gilles de la Tourette. In: Georges Gilles de la Tourette: Beyond the eponym. Oxford: Oxford University Press 2018; 337–51.

Walusinski O. Théophraste Renaudot (1586–1653): Gilles de la Tourette's hero. In: Georges Gilles de la Tourette: Beyond the eponym. Oxford: Oxford University Press 2018; 353–69.

Walusinski O. Commentator for La revue hebdomadaire, 1892–1900. In: Georges Gilles de la Tourette: Beyond the eponym. Oxford: Oxford University Press 2018; 371–90.

Walusinski O. Correspondence between Octave Lebesgue, known as Georges Montorgueil, and Gilles de la Tourette. In: Georges Gilles de la Tourette: Beyond the eponym. Oxford: Oxford University Press 2018; 391–412.

Walusinski O. Gilles de la Tourette the poet? In: Georges Gilles de la Tourette: Beyond the eponym. Oxford: Oxford University Press 2018; 413–17.

Walusinski O. Recapitulative list of all Gilles de la Tourette's publications. In: Georges Gilles de la Tourette: Beyond the eponym. Oxford: Oxford University Press 2018; 421–62.

Websites

European Society for the Study of Tourette Syndrome (ESSTS): www.essts.org

Tourettes Action – UK: http://tourettes-action.org.uk

Tourette Association of America (TAA): www.tourette.org

Index